THE INADEQUATE LUTEAL PHASE

THE INADEQUATE LUTEAL PHASE

PATHOPHYSIOLOGY, DIAGNOSTICS, THERAPY

Edited by
H.-D. Taubert
and H. Kuhl

The Proceedings of the Seventh Freiburg Colloquium, a Serono
Workshop on Reproductive Medicine held at Freiburg/Breisgau,
September 1983

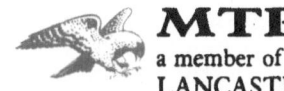 **MTP PRESS LIMITED**
a member of the KLUWER ACADEMIC PUBLISHERS GROUP
LANCASTER / BOSTON / THE HAGUE / DORDRECHT

Published in the UK and Europe by
MTP Press Limited
Falcon House
Lancaster, England

British Library Cataloguing in Publication Data

Serono Workshop on Reproductive Medicine
 1983: Freiburg/Breisgau
 The inadequate luteal phase.
 1. Corpus luteum—Diseases
 I. Title   II. Taubert, H.-D.   III. Kuhl, H.
 618.1'1   RG441
 ISBN 978-94-015-7164-7   ISBN 978-94-015-7162-3 (eBook)
 DOI 10.1007/978-94-015-7162-3
Published in the USA by
MTP Press
A division of Kluwer Boston Inc
190 Old Derby Street
Hingham, MA 02043, USA

Library of Congress Cataloging in Publication Data

Main entry under title:

The Inadequate luteal phase.

  "Proceedings of the Seventh Freiburg Colloquium . . .
1983."
  Bibliography: p.
  Includes index.
  1. Luteal phase defects—Congresses.   I. Taubert,
H. D. (Hans-Dieter), 1931–   .   II. Kuhl, H. (Herbert),
1940–   .   III. Freiburg Colloquium on Reproductive
Medicine (7th: 1983)
RG205.L87153   1984   618.1'78   84-4379

Phototypesetting by Blackpool Typesetting Services Ltd.
132 Highfield Road, Blackpool, England.

Contents

CONTENTS

List of Participants

Dr. med. SUSANNE BAUMGARTEN
Abteilung für gynäkologische
  Endokrinologie, Sterilität und
  Familienplanung
Klinikum Steglitz der Freien Universität
Hindenburgdamm 30
D-1000 Berlin 45
F.R. Germany

Prof. Dr. med. GERHARD BETTENDORF
Abteilung für klinische und experimentelle
  Endokrinologie
Universitäts-Frauenklinik
Martinistraße 52
D-2000 Hamburg
F.R. Germany

Prof. Dr. med. WILHELM BRAENDLE
Abteilung für klinische und experimentelle
  Endokrinologie
Universitäts-Frauenklinik
Martinistraße 52
D-2000 Hamburg
F.R. Germany

Prof. Dr. med. MEINERT BRECKWOLDT
Direktor der Abteilung für gynäkologische
  Endokrinologie
Universitäts-Frauenklinik
Hugstetter Straße 55
D-7800 Freiburg-Breisgau
F.R. Germany

Prof. Dr. med. GISELA
  DALLENBACH-HELLWEG
Institut für Pathologie
A2, 2.
D-6800 Mannheim 1
F.R. Germany

Prof. Dr. med. ERHARD DAUME
Abteilung für gynäkologische
  Endokrinologie und Reproduktion
Zentrum für Frauenheilkunde und
  Geburtshilfe
Philipps-Universität
Pilgrimsteine 3
D-3550 Marburg
F.R. Germany

Dr. phil. nat. JEANNE SIOE ENG
  DERICKS-TAN
Abteilung für gynäkologische
  Endokrinologie
Universitäts-Frauenklinik
J. W. Goethe-Universität
Theodor-Stern-Kai 7
D-6000 Frankfurt am Main 70
F.R. Germany

Dr. med. GABRIELE GAHN
Universitäts-Frauenklinik
J. W. Goethe-Universität
Theodor-Stern-Kai 7
D-6000 Frankfurt am Main 70
F.R. Germany

Prof. JEAN GAUTRAY
Faculté de Médecine de CRETEIL
  (Univ. Paris XII)
Obstètrique–Gynécologic CHIC
F-94010 Creteil Cédex
France

Dr. med. FRANZ GEISTHÖVEL
  Wissenschaftlicher Assistent
Abteilung für gynäkologische
  Endokrinologie
Universitäts-Frauenklinik
Hugstetter Straße 55
D-7800 Freiburg-Breisgau
F.R. Germany

vii

Priv.-Doz. Dr. med. INGRID GERHARD
Abteilung für gynäkologische
 Endokrinologie
Universitäts-Frauenklinik
Voßstraße 9
D-6900 Heidelberg
F.R. Germany

Prof. Dr. VACLAV INSLER
Division of Obstetrics and Gynecology
Soroka Medical Center
P.O.B. 151
Beer-Sheba
Israel

Prof. Dr. med. PAUL J. KELLER
Departement für Frauenheilkunde–
 Endokrinologie
Frauenklinikstraße 10
CH-8091 Zürich
Switzerland

Dr. med. ROSEMARIE KÖHLER
Frauenklinik der Westfälischen
Wilhelms-Universität
Dogmagkstraße 11/D
D-4400 Münster
F.R. Germany

Dr. PHILIPPE KONINCKX
Academic Hospital St. Raphael
Gasthuisberg
Katholicke Universiteit Leuven
B-3000 Leuven
Belgium

Prof. Dr. phil. nat. HERBERT KUHL
Abteilung für gynäkologische
 Endokrinologie
Universitäts-Frauenklinik
J. W. Goethe-Universität
Theodor-Stern-Kai 7
D-6000 Frankfurt am Main 70
F.R. Germany

Prof. Dr. med. FRANK LEHMANN
Universitäts-Frauenklinik
Ratzeburger Allee 160
D-2400 Lübeck
F.R. Germany

Dr. MARC L'HERMITE
Université Libre de Bruxelles
Unité d'Endocrinologie Sexuelle
Dept. of Obstetrics and Gynecology
Hôpital Universitaire Brugman
Place A. van Gehuchten 4
B-1020 Bruxelles
Belgium

Dr. med. JOSEF MUSIL
Medizinischer Direktor
Serono GmbH
Merzhauser Straße 134
D-7800 Freiburg/Breisgau
F.R. Germany

Prof. IRVING ROTHCHILD
Department of Reproductive Biology
Case Western Reserve University School
 of Medicine
2105 Adelbert Road
Cleveland, OH 44106
USA

Prof. Dr. med. BENNO RUNNEBAUM
Frauenklinik, Abteilung 8.1.2.
Gynäkologische Endokrinologie
Voßstraße 9
D-6900 Heidelberg
F.R. Germany

Prof. Dr. med. H. P. G. SCHNEIDER
Frauenklinik der Westfälischen
Wilhelms Universität
Domagkstraße 11/D
D-4400 Münster
F.R. Germany

Priv.-Doz. Dr. med. K.-W. SCHWEPPE
Frauenklinik der Westfälischen
Wilhelms-Universität
Domagkstraße 11/D
D-4400 Münster
F.R. Germany

**Prof. Dr. med. HANS-DIETER
 TAUBERT**
Abteilung für gynäkologische
 Endokrinologie
Universitäts-Frauenklinik
J. W. Goethe-Universität
Theodor-Stern-Kai 7
D-6000 Frankfurt am Main 70
F.R. Germany

Prof. ANNE COLSTON WENTZ
Department of Obstetrics and Gynecology
Director, Division of Reproductive
 Endocrinology
Director, Center for Fertility and
 Reproductive Research
Vanderbilt University Medical Center
Nashville, TN 37232
USA

Preface

The idea of holding a 2-day workshop on such a narrow topic as the *inadequate luteal phase* evolved out of a certain sense of dismay of the clinician about being confronted in daily practice by an entity which does not cause any noticeable symptoms, although it keeps women from bearing children, evades a clear diagnostic classification, as its causes are difficult to grasp, and often resists treatment for no obvious reasons, even though some women conceive without having been treated.

The aim of this workshop was to provide a number of clinical and basic scientists from several European countries, Israel, and the USA with an opportunity to review the current state of knowledge on luteal phase inadequacy, and to make an attempt at defining some principles for future diagnostic and therapeutic approaches. It would have been unrealistic to expect this workshop to provide a solution for every unsolved problem. It is hoped, however, that the expertise of the members of this panel brought about some clarification of disputed issues, helped to dispatch some time-honoured concepts which had outlived their usefulness, and to take the first careful steps in treading new ground.

We would like to thank all the speakers, their co-workers, the chairpersons, and the discussants for their contributions which helped to make this a very lively workshop. Our particular gratitude is due to Mr Rainer Felbiert, Director of Serono Pharmaceuticals, Freiburg/Breisgau, F.R. Germany, and Dr med. Josef Musil, Medical Director, without whose engagement and wholesome support this workshop could not have been conducted as the VIIth Freiburg Colloquium on Reproductive Medicine. We would also like to thank Mrs Maria Luigia Wiegand and Mrs Monika Schwär for expertly taking care of organizational matters.

Frankfurt am Main, 20 October, 1983   *Hans-Dieter Taubert*
Herbert Kuhl

Introduction: luteal phase inadequacy: a quest for new insights

H.-D. TAUBERT

Since *luteal phase inadequacy* was first described by Jones[1] in 1949 as a cause of functional infertility and of first trimester abortion, a large amount of information has been accumulated supporting the notion that the aetiology of this entity is rather heterogeneous.

Being by definition a disorder of the ovulatory cycle, luteal phase inadequacy is characterized by incomplete or delayed secretory transformation of the endometrium rendering it as a poor substrate for the implantation of the blastocyst. The faulty secretory transformation of the endometrium is usually attributed to a malfunction of the corpus luteum, or to an inherent defect of the endometrium[2]. It appears to be particularly prevalent in women suffering repeated abortions[3,4], in premenopausal, still-ovulating patients[5], and subsequent to ovulation-induction with clomiphene[6,7]. In addition, a variety of other possible causes for subnormal secretion of progesterone has been described: delayed onset of luteinization[8], inadequate stimulation by LH[9-12], interference with the function of the corpus luteum by intermittent or moderate hyperprolactinaemia[13-18], or hyperandrogenaemia[19], and – possibly in a substantial number of cases – improper follicular maturation subsequent to a relative FSH deficit in the early follicular phase[8,20,21].

While reviewing the medical records of 484 patients with primary and secondary infertility who had been under my care during the years from 1968 to 1978, a rather startling observation was made, in that not less than 168 out of 368 patients who completed the basic work-up and entered into the stage of therapy – and had not become pregnant prior to the completion of the diagnostic work-up, as 37 out of the remaining 116 women did – had been diagnosed as suffering from luteal phase inadequacy (45.6%). This meant that luteal phase inadequacy was diagnosed more often than anovulation (33.2%), and both exceeded every other cause of infertility to a large degree (Haiges, P. and Taubert, H.-D., unpublished results). Even though this group of women was certainly preselected and not representative for the general infertile population, in that most of these patients had been referred by practising gynaecologists to the Infertility Clinic after having already undergone more or less extensive treatment, this percentage was clearly much higher than previous estimates in the literature, which ranged from 0.4% to approximately 10%[22]. This unusually high incidence raised the question whether this pathological entity, or whatever is labelled by the term luteal phase inadequacy or its numerous synonyms (e.g. short luteal phase, corpus luteum defect, luteal phase insufficiency or defect, cycle insufficiency), tends to occur more often than before, is recognized more readily as a consequence of greater awareness, or was simply over-diagnosed. The latter possibility also raised some doubt as to whether the currently used diagnostic criteria suffice for distinguishing between a normal and abnormal luteal phase.

It has been our policy to consider an atypical basal body temperature record merely as an indicator for the presence of an inadequate luteal phase, and to base the diagnosis primarily upon the result of an endometrial biopsy taken shortly before the onset of menstruation.

As a fair number of patients with the histological finding of *endometrial inadequacy* conceives, however, and eventually carries to term without having been treated, the information gained from a finding of incomplete secretory transformation of the endometrium and its pathognomonic significance appears to be debatable unless one subscribes to the notion that luteal phase inadequacy does not have to manifest itself in all cycles. This, of course, re-opens the search for an answer to the question as to what actually causes a luteal phase to be inadequate with respect to supporting the development of the earliest stages of pregnancy.

Although it has been our experience that the assessment of endometrial biopsies is not improved by the application of histochemical techniques[23], ultrastructural studies may provide us with new insight into the underlying pathological processes at the level of the endometrium.

If, on the other hand, the secretory capacity of the corpus luteum were always affected, *luteal inadequacy* could readily be discovered by measuring serum progesterone, and this should then be preferred to an endometrial biopsy. Even though peripheral blood levels of progesterone may reflect the secretory capacity of the corpus luteum, there is reason to believe that in some cases there may be a marked discrepancy between serum progesterone and endometrial development[24]. This circumstance should be seriously considered before a plea is made to abandon the endometrial biopsy altogether.

As the application of the presently used diagnostic methods has reached a certain impasse, it will be one of the most interesting aspects of this workshop to discuss the possible merits of sonography in diagnosing and following the therapy of luteal phase inadequacy.

The problem of diagnosing luteal phase inadequacy properly has been confounded by the fact that this entity quite often does not seem to be a constant phenomenon, but rather a facet of a pathological process of varying intensity which may manifest itself in manifold ways, and vacillate in a wide spectrum ranging from frank anovulation to the syndrome of the luteinized, unruptured follicle[8, 25], to luteal phase inadequacy, and eventually to the normal ovulatory cycle. The recognition of this still ill-understood and poorly defined entity may be improved by a better understanding of the role of prolactin, gonadotropins, androgens, inhibin and other follicular inhibiting substances, and by the rational use of function tests such as the metoclopramide-, LH–RH-, and hCG-test.

INTRODUCTION

The value of animal models which are available for the study of luteal phase inadequacy remains questionable, as there are considerable differences in the regulation of human corpus luteum function. Therefore, studies on the performance of the corpus luteum after follicle aspiration may also aid our understanding of the pathogenesis of disturbed luteal function.

We are faced with a similar dilemma with respect to therapy, in that there are as yet no valid guidelines as to whether to use progesterone or synthetic progestogens as a first treatment of choice, or to stimulate the function of the corpus luteum directly or indirectly by the use of hCG or ovulation-inducers. It has been our experience that hCG, clomiphene, and dydro-gesterone gave similar rates of success when applied as a first method of choice, and that a change to another therapeutic agent was almost equally effective in each group. As a fair number of women with luteal phase inadequacy becomes pregnant without having been treated with hormonal preparations, the effectiveness and specificity of such therapy has to be questioned. This is supported by the fact that, irrespective of the type of therapy used, the pregnancy and birth rates quoted in many reports neither convince nor satisfy. A radical change in such an unsatisfactory situation is not likely to occur until we begin to understand better what makes a luteal phase inadequate. It would be preposterous to expect the VIIth Freiburg Colloquium on Reproductive Medicine to succeed in solving all the riddles posed by this enigmatic and elusive cause of infertility. It is our hope, however, that the presentation of new scientific material, laboratory data, and clinical observations, and its discussion by this panel, will provide us with a better understanding of the problems of luteal phase inadequacy.

References

1. Jones, G. S. (1949). Some newer aspects of the management of infertility. *J. Am. Med. Assoc.*, **141**, 1123
2. Keller, D. W., Wiest, W. G., Askin, F. B., Johnson, L. W. and Strickler, R. C. (1979). Pseudocorpus luteum insufficiency: a local defect of progesterone action on endometrial tissue. *J. Clin. Endocrinol. Metab.*, **48**, 127
3. McDonough, P. G., Tho, P. T. and Byrd, J. R. (1978). Evaluation of reproductive failure in 101 couples. *Fertil. Steril.*, **30** (Suppl.), 720.
4. Grant, A., McBride, W. G. and Moyes, J. M. (1959). Luteal phase defects in abortion. *Int. J. Fertil.*, **4**, 323
5. Sherman, B. M. and Korenman, S. G. (1975). Hormonal characteristics of the human menstrual cycle throughout reproductive life. *J. Clin. Invest.*, **55**, 699
6. Garcia, J., Jones, G. S. and Wentz, A. C. (1977). The use of clomiphene citrate. *Fertil. Steril.*, **37**, 755
7. van Hall, E. V. and Mastboom, J. L. (1969). Luteal phase insufficiency in patients treated with clomiphene. *Am. J. Obstet. Gynecol.*, **103**, 165
8. Koninckx, P. R., Heyns, W. J., Corvelyn, P. and Brosens, I. A. (1978). Delayed onset of luteinization as a cause of infertility. *Fertil. Steril.*, **29**, 266
9. Dreykluft, R., Magnus, U., Zielske, F. and Hammerstein, J. (1971). Normal and disturbed function of the human corpus luteum as reflected by hormonal analysis in blood. *Acta Endocrinol. (Copenh.)*, **152** (Suppl.), 69
10. Jürgensen, O., Hildebrandt, H., Fritz, I., Kronauer, J. and Taubert, H.-D. (1973). Plasma LH und Progesteron in normalen und gestörten Zyklen. *Arch. Gynaekol.*, **214**, 418

11. van de Kerckhove, D. and Dhont, M. (1972). The relationship between serum LH levels, as determined by radioimmunoassay, and the life span of the corpus luteum. *Ann. Endocrinol.*, **33**, 205

12. Lepoutre, L., Dhont, M. and van de Kerckhove, D. (1973). LH and progesterone in the menstrual cycle: further observations with the length of the luteal phase. *Ann. Endocrinol.*, **34**, 327.

13. Coelingh-Bennink, H. J. T. (1979). Intermittent bromocriptine treatment for the induction of ovulation in hyperprolactinemia. *Fertil. Steril.*, **31**, 267

14. Seppälä, M., Hirvonen, E. and Ranta, T. (1976). Hyperprolactinemia and luteal insufficiency. *Lancet*, **1**, 229

15. Mühlenstedt, D., Meissner, M. and Schneider, H. P. G. (1979). Short luteal phase and prolactin. *Int. J. Fertil.*, **23**, 213

16. Del Pozo, E., Wyss, H., Alcaniz, J., Campana, A. and Naftolin, F. (1979). Prolactin and deficient luteal function. *Obstet. Gynecol.*, **53**, 282

17. Saunders, D. M., Hunter, J. C., Haase, H. R. and Wilson, G. R. (1979). Treatment of luteal phase inadequacy with bromocriptine. *Obstet. Gynecol.*, **53**, 287

18. Mühlenstedt, D., Meissner, M. and Schneider, H. P. G. (1979). Prolactin and luteal phase defect. *Geburtshilfe Frauenheilkd.*, **39**, 580

19. Rodriguez-Rigau, L. J., Smith, K. D., Tcholakian, R. K. and Steinberger, E. (1979). Effect of prednisone on plasma testosterone levels and on duration of phases of the menstrual cycle in hyperandrogenic women. *Fertil. Steril.*, **32**, 408

20. Di Zerega, G. S. and Hodgen, G. D. (1981). Luteal phase dysfunction: A sequel to aberrant folliculogenesis. *Fertil. Steril.*, **35**, 489

21. Strott, C. A., Cargille, C. M., Ross, G. T. and Lipsett, M. B. (1970). The short luteal phase. *J. Clin. Endocrinol. Metab.*, **30**, 246

22. Taubert, H.-D. (1978). Luteal phase insufficiency. In Keller, P. J. (ed.) *Contr. Gynecol. Obstet.*, vol. 4, pp. 78–113. (Basel: S. Karger)

23. Geisz, J. (1976). Histochemische, hormonale und autoradiographische Untersuchungen beim Lutealphasendefekt. (Frankfurt am Main: Inaugural-Dissertation)

24. Perez, R. J., Plurad, A. V. and Palladion, V. S. (1981). The relationship of the corpus luteum and the endometrium in infertile patients. *Fertil. Steril.*, **35**, 423

25. Marik, J. and Hulka, J. (1978). Luteinized unruptured follicle syndrome: a subtle cause of infertility. *Fertil. Steril.*, **29**, 270

Section 1
Pathogenesis

1
Follicular development and ovarian inhibitors

E. DAUME, S. CHARI AND T. HILLENSJOE

INTRODUCTION

It is now well recognized that the maturation of a follicle up to the stage of ovulation depends on stimulation by adequate amounts of FSH and LH in appropriate proportions[1-3]. In the immature ovarian follicle the granulosa cell is the target for FSH, whereas LH acts primarily upon the theca cell. FSH stimulation brings about an increase in the steroidogenic potential of the granulosa cells (i.e. estrogen production), an induction of granulosa cell LH receptors, and an enhancement of granulosa cell aromatase activity[3, 4]. LH acts on the theca cells to provide the androgen substrate which can be aromatized in the granulosa cells to estrogens[5]. The acquisition of aromatizing enzyme which regulates the biosynthesis of estrogens from androgenic precursors appears, therefore, to be a critical factor for the selection of a preovulatory follicle[6].

Although many follicles undergo a certain amount of growth and development during the reproductive cycle of mammals, only a certain number eventually reaches the stage of ovulation, while the rest becomes atretic. Several concepts have been proposed to explain the process of atresia[7]. Even though all follicles are exposed to the same extraovarian regulators, e.g. LH and FSH, there are considerable differences in the microenvironment of individual follicles[8-11]. It has been shown that healthy follicles invariably have an elevated estrogen to androgen ratio, whereas the reverse relationship is found in atretic follicles[3, 9].

If atresia is due to differences in aromatizing capacity, it may actually be caused by different degrees of sensitivity of follicles towards gonadotropins. It has indeed been suggested[4] that none of the follicles present at the beginning of a menstrual cycle which has the potential to reach the pre-ovulatory stage will attain full maturation unless it has been exposed sufficiently to the action of FSH to pass a critical threshold. This 'threshold' is apparently determined for each follicle by one or more variables such as (a) local vascularization optimizing the accessibility of follicles to gonadotropins[12],

(b) the number of follicular granulosa cells and/or gonadotropin receptors per cell which would determine a differential response to gonadotropins[3], and (c) interfollicular levels of substances which modulate the action of gonadotropins *per se*[4, 12].

As some of these possible pathways have already been reviewed elsewhere[4, 12, 13], especially with respect to steroids and LH–RH-like intraovarian factors, we would like to discuss in some detail the non-steroidal factors which have as yet been proven, or at least been postulated, to exist in the follicular fluid: inhibin/folliculostatin, oocyte maturation inhibitor (OMI), follicle-stimulating hormone-binding inhibitor (FSH-BI), luteinization inhibitor (LI), and luteinization stimulator (LS).

INHIBIN

It is generally accepted that ovarian steroid hormones modulate the release of pituitary gonadotropins as originally postulated 50 years ago by Moore and Price[14], Hohlweg and Junkmann[15], and Hohlweg[16]. The modulation involves inhibitory (negative) and stimulatory (positive) feedback effects exerted at the level of both the hypothalamus and pituitary. Recent experimental and circumstantial evidence suggests the existence of a second negative feedback regulator of pituitary gonadotropin secretion which has been called inhibin[17–19]. Whether the action of inhibin is specific for the regulation of FSH release is still a matter of controversy. Our own studies with human follicular fluid inhibin indicate that the specificity of its action depends upon the physiological state of experimental animals.

We demonstrated the existence of two molecular species with inhibin activity in human follicular fluid (hFF), i.e. big inhibin designated as UF

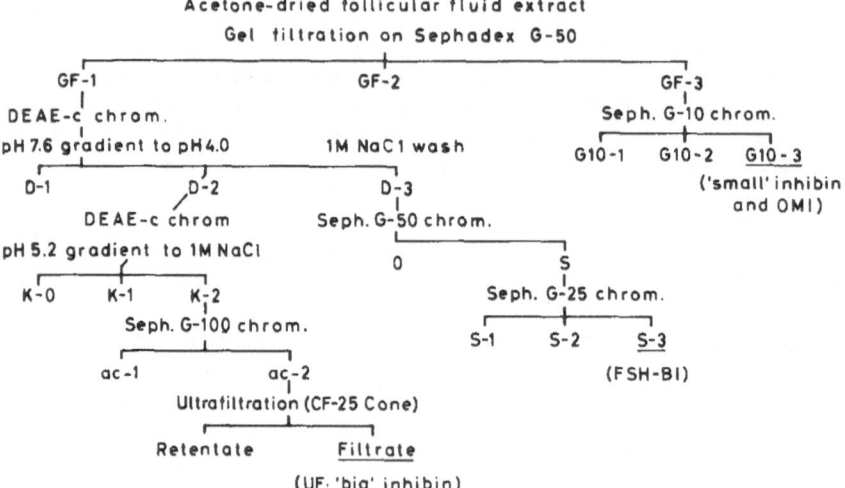

Figure 1.1 Flow diagram: steps used for purification of big inhibin, small inhibin (OMI) and FSH-BI

(ultra-filtrate) with a molecular weight of 23 000, and small inhibin (GF-3/G-10-3) which has a MW of < 1000. The flow diagram (Figure 1.1) delineates the steps for the purification of the active principles. Details have been published elsewhere[20–22].

BIOLOGICAL CHARACTERISTICS OF BIG INHIBIN

Inhibin as a feedback-signal

Highly purified big inhibin selectively suppressed FSH secretion by rat hemipituitaries *in vitro* (Figure 1.2). It also inhibited, *in vivo*, the specific rise in FSH and subsequent ovarian compensatory hypertrophy following unilateral ovariectomy in rats[22, 23].

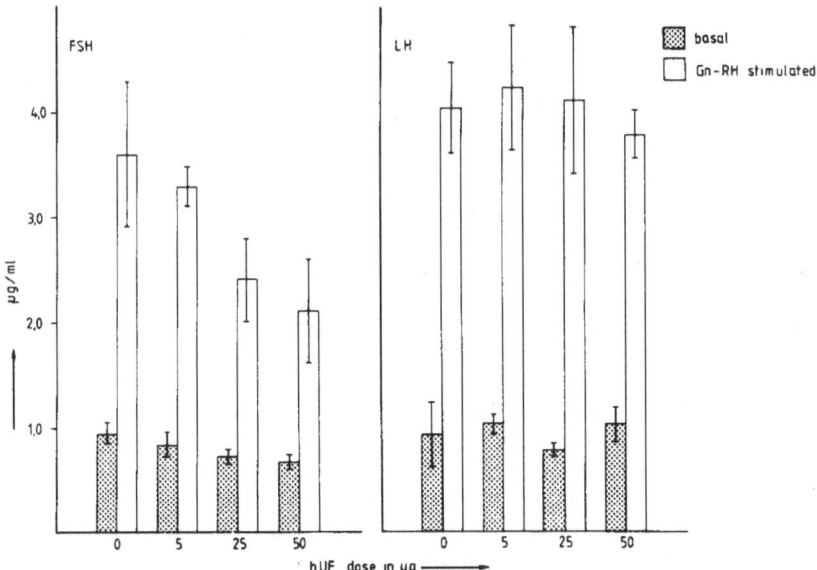

Figure 1.2 Effect of hFF–big inhibin on pituitary gonadotropin secretion *in vitro*. Pituitaries were recovered from 40 to 44 days old male rats and bisected. Two hemipituitaries per tube incubated in MEM (supplemented with 10 mmol/l HEPES and 100 μg/ml penicillin/streptomycin) at 37 °C. One hour later the medium was withdrawn, fresh medium containing GnRH (4 ng/ml per tube) was added and incubated for a further 3 h. FSH and LH in the media were determined by RIA using NIAMDD kits

Kraulis *et al.*[24, 25] demonstrated that in sexually immature female rats a precocious surge of LH and FSH can be induced by sex steroids provided that animals have previously been exposed to an estrogen. We found that pretreatment of such estrogen-primed rats with big inhibin highly significantly inhibited the LH-surge induced by progesterone[21, 22]. In an earlier study, hFF-inhibin has been shown to suppress both the basal and the GnRH-induced release of LH in experimentally cryptorchidized rats[26]. These data

9

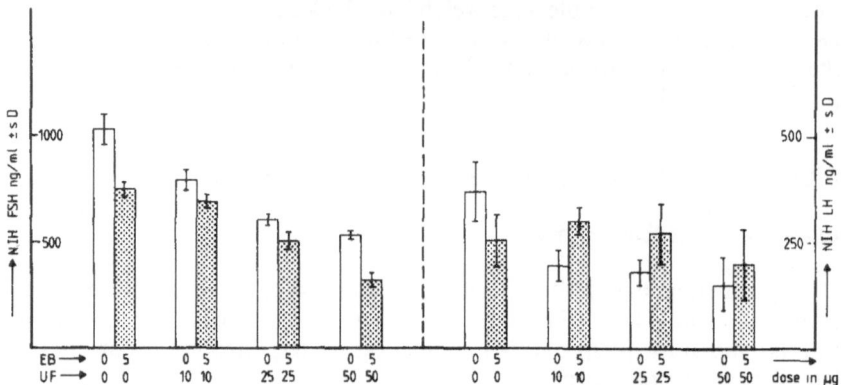

Figure 1.3 Effect of simultaneous treatment *in vivo* with estradiol benzoate (EB) and big inhibin on serum FSH and LH. Adult female rats were ovariectomized. On day 7 after surgery groups of rats were treated with saline/EB (controls), big inhibin (UF) and inhibin plus EB. The total dose of inhibin was injected intraperitoneally thrice at 12 h intervals and EB (5 µg/100 g body-weight) administered subcutaneously as a single injection just prior to the first injection of inhibin. FSH and LH were estimated by RIA.

provide a reasonable basis for the assumption that the regulation of both FSH and LH secretion is an intrinsic property of inhibin.

It has also been observed that the negative feedback effect of big inhibin is more pronounced in the presence of steroids. In adult ovariectomized (OVX) rats, when injected alone, it diminished the peripheral levels of FSH and LH. When administered to OVX, estrogen-primed rats, the inhibition of FSH was increased, while there was no significant change in the level of LH (Figure 1.3). Bronson and Channing[27] observed that a variety of steroids failed to suppress FSH in maximally estrogenized OVX mice, while steroid-free porcine follicular fluid (pFF) as well as mouse ovarian homogenates, exerted an additive suppressive effect. A seemingly high dose of 100 ml pFF had to be given to OVX monkeys[18] to suppress plasma FSH to the baseline, whereas in intact animals as little as 5 ml given daily for 3 days during the follicular phase sufficed to suppress FSH to or below the lowest level observed at any time throughout the menstrual cycle.

These observations indicate an interaction of ovarian steroids and inhibin in the regulation of gonadotropin secretion. As big inhibin has been shown to inhibit the secretion of GnRH by rat hypothalami *in vitro*[21,22], it may be assumed that the hypothalamus is also under the influence of a feedback effect of inhibin. This concept receives further support from a recent report of Condon *et al.*[29] These authors could show that the injection of a steroid-free extract of pFF into OVX rats bearing estrogen-containing silastic capsules blocked the primary surge of FSH. The same effect could be brought about by the direct application of the pFF extract to the dorsal anterior hypothalamic area by means of chronically implanted cannulas. This suggests that ovarian inhibin acts at least in part at the level of the central nervous system.

Inhibin as a regulator of intraovarian function

The possible significance of inhibin in the regulation of intraovarian function is worth considering, as several observations made with big inhibin suggest such a role. The administration of the inhibitor into female rats daily for 10 days beginning on day 10 after birth resulted in structural alterations of the ovary leading to atresia in spite of concomitant treatment with human menopausal gonadotropin (hMG)[29]. Furthermore, inhibin diminished the hMG-induced estrogen secretion (E_2), and increased the testosterone (T) levels[22]. At this stage it is difficult to explain the possible mechanism of action of inhibin in inducing atresia. The suppression of endogenous FSH alone cannot well account for the changes in the micro-environment in the ovary, since the administration of exogenous gonadotropin (hMG) could not overcome the influence of inhibin. On the other hand, the decrease of E_2 levels in these rats with a parallel increase in T is indicative of a possible inhibition of aromatization of T by inhibin. In this context, a recent report of Hillier et al.[4] is of interest. They observed that in the rat granulosa-cell culture model, bovine follicular fluid (bFF), and the fractions thereof containing FSH-BI or inhibin activity all inhibited the induction of aromatase activity in proportion to their concentration in the culture medium. Recently, DiZerega et al.[30] have identified proteins (MW range 14 000–18 000) secreted by the dominant human follicle, which were capable of inhibiting hMG-induced ovarian weight increase as well as diminishing serum E_2 levels in 23-day-old, hypophysectomized, diethylstilboestrol-treated rats.

In immature rats, treatment with pregnant mare serum gonadotropin (PMSG) induces the development of preovulatory follicles which respond to an ovulatory dose of hCG. One of the hCG-induced reactions in these animals is an increase in progesterone synthesis by granulosa cells[31]. Pretreatment of 24–25-day-old, hMG-primed rats with hFF-inhibin brought about a highly significant inhibition of the hCG-induced progesterone secretion[22]. Two modes of action may be proposed to explain this effect. Firstly, treatment with inhibin may interfere with the action of hMG in inducing the development of preovulatory follicles. Although no histological examination was performed in this study, the lack of difference in ovarian weight between the controls and treated animals renders this possibility unlikely.

On the other hand, pretreatment with inhibin alters the preovulatory follicle in such a way that it cannot synthesize progesterone (P) in response to hCG. Further experimentation will be necessary to determine whether inhibin affects the process of ovulation by either or both mechanisms.

SMALL INHIBIN (GF-3/G-10-3)

This moiety was separated from hFF by chromatography on Sephadex G-50 followed by Sephadex G-10 (Figure 1.1). The chemical nature of this fraction has not yet been established[21]. Inhibin activity was demonstrated in this fraction in a dose range of 0.5–5.0 µg in vivo, and 0.05–2.0 µg in vitro[21].

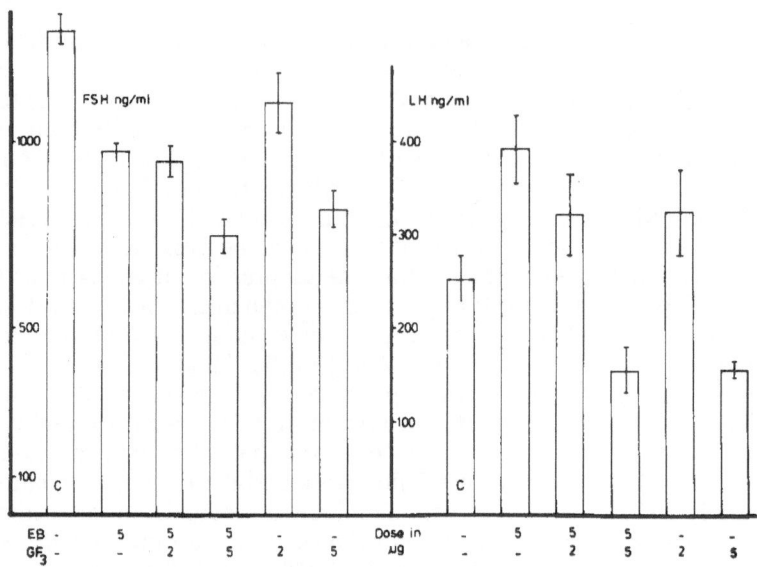

Figure 1.4 Effect of simultaneous treatment *in vivo* with EB and small inhibin on serum FSH and LH. For conditions refer to Figure 1.3

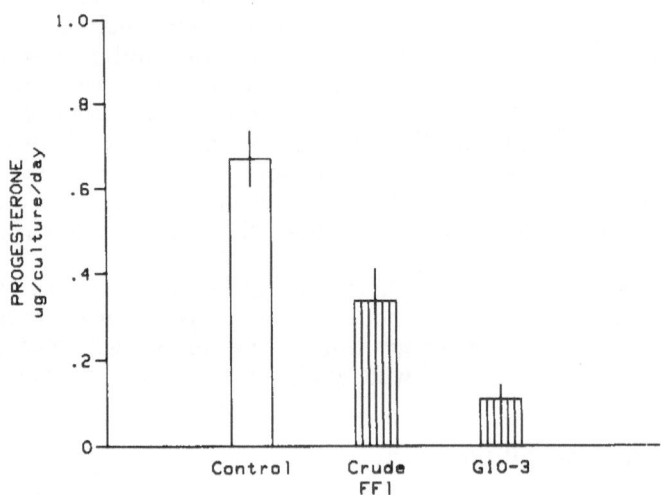

Figure 1.5 Progesterone accumulation in granulosa cells obtained from a 22 mm follicle on day 16 of the cycle. The patient had been treated with clomiphene followed by hCG (4500 IU) 35 h before operation. Mean ± SE of duplicate cell cultures are shown. The dose of the crude, lyophilized FF1 was 5 mg/ml, and that of G10-3 was 150 µg/ml. Culture period: 0–2 days

Unlike big inhibin, this fraction showed neither additive nor synergistic effects in suppressing gonadotropin levels in OVX, estrogenized rats (Figure 1.4). As in the case of big inhibin, chronic treatment of 10-day-old rats for 10 days with hMG and G-10-3 inhibited the hMG-induced rise in serum E_2 levels. In addition, the fraction G-10-3 was also found to be capable of blocking the hCG-induced surge of progesterone in 25-day-old, hMG-primed rats (unpublished results). Interestingly, *in vitro* tests revealed that both GF-3 and G-10-3 could inhibit the maturation of rat oocytes as well as the secretion of P by rat and human granulosa cells[32, 33]. At certain concentrations, this GF-3 fraction could also inhibit the binding of FSH to porcine granulosa cells *in vitro*[21].

OOCYTE MATURATION INHIBITOR (OMI)

The observation that an oocyte, under physiological conditions, does not undergo the maturation division before ovulation led to the assumption that the follicular fluid contains an oocyte maturation inhibiting factor[18]. OMI from porcine follicular fluid (pFF) has been partially purified[34-36], and appears to be a peptide with a mass of less than 2000. Some effects of OMI have been determined *in vitro*. It reversibly inhibits the spontaneous maturation of isolated pig oocytes, and also the P secretion by cumulus cells[37]. The effect on meiotic divisions was not species specific[38]. The existence of OMI activity in human follicular fluid was first demonstrated by Hillensjoe *et al.*[39].

The report on OMI having a molecular weight of less than 2000 prompted us to examine the small inhibin (GF-3/G-10-3) purified by chromatography on Sephadex G-50 and G-10 (Figure 1.1) for OMI activity. We observed that this fraction could reversibly inhibit meiosis in oocytes with cumulus as well as denuded ones isolated from the preovulatory follicles of PSMG-treated, immature rats[32]. It also inhibited reversibly P secretion by cumulus and mural granulosa cells *in vitro*[32, 40]. Evidence has also been presented that this molecule inhibits P secretion by human granulosa cells in culture (Figure 1.5)[33].

FOLLICLE-STIMULATING HORMONE BINDING INHIBITOR (FSH-BI)

Ovarian function is regulated not only by circulating levels of gonadotropins, but also by the presence or absence, at the appropriate physiological sites, of factors capable of regulating the binding of the hormones to their receptors. Darga and Reichert[41] first reported on the presence of a small molecular weight substance in bFF capable of inhibiting the binding of radiolabelled hFSH to granulosa cells *in vitro*. Evidence for the existence of a factor with FSH-BI activity in hFF was presented by Daume *et al.*[42]. Partially purified FSH-BI activity from hFF (Figure 1.1) with a molecular weight of approximately 1200 d, inhibited in a dose-related manner the binding of iodinated hFSH to porcine granulosa cells *in vitro*[43].

It must be emphasized, however, that the presence of small molecular weight inhibitors in not unique to the follicular fluid. For example, FSH-BI activity has also been isolated from human serum[44], human ovarian cyst fluid, and ascites. Sephadex gel chromatography of serum samples obtained from post-menopausal women, cows, and ovariectomized rats indicated the presence of small inhibin/OMI-*like* factor. When tested by bioassay, however, neither inhibin nor OMI-like activity could be located in this fraction[21,32].

LUTEINIZATION INHIBITOR (LI) AND LUTEINIZATION STIMULATOR (LS)

pFF obtained from small follicles has been shown to contain a factor which inhibits spontaneous luteinization of granulosa cells, progesterone secretion, prostaglandin F_2 secretion, responsiveness to LH, FSH, prostaglandin E_1 and E_2, FSH-binding, RNA synthesis, and adenyl cyclase activity[45]. The absence of such an inhibitor in large follicles led to the speculation that as the follicle matures it either loses the inhibitory activity or gains a substance that enhances luteinization (LS).

The stimulatory actions of follicular fluid on granulosa cells include: morphological maturation, progesterone and estrogen secretion, enhanced responsiveness to gonadotropins and activation of ornithin decarboxylase. LI activity has been found in fractions representing a molecular weight of less, and more, than 10 000, respectively. It is resistant to heating at 60 °C, but is unstable at 80 °C.

Contrary to that, LS activity has only been found in the MW > 10 000 fraction, partially purified by ultrafiltration and column chromatography[45]. Channing et al.[18] have reported that both LI and LS activities are present to some extent in follicles at various stages of maturation, and they suggest that the changing ratio of LS/LI (or the lack of a change) may modulate the response of individual follicles to circulating gonadotropins. However, any definite conclusions regarding the physiological role of LS and LI in the regulation of follicular maturation should be deferred until the results of studies with chemically pure substances are available.

DISCUSSION

It has become evident that the regulation of follicular maturation, i.e. growth and steroidogenesis, and oocyte maturation depend upon an interaction between pituitary gonadotropins and follicular steroidal and non-steroidal factors.

DiZerega et al.[46] have shown that the normal time course of development and endocrine function of the follicle depends on the exposure of the ovary to a normal, tonic stimulation by FSH during the perimenstrual period and follicular phase of the cycle. The finding of spontaneous luteal inadequacy being associated with abnormal FSH secretion in both women[47] and monkeys[48] also indicates that the control of the action of FSH upon the ovary is essential for normal reproductive function.

The polycystic ovary syndrome is characterized by an inappropriate secretion of gonadotropins, i.e. a high basal LH to FSH ratio[48, 50]. Tanabe *et al.*[51] speculate on the basis of their observations that elevated levels of LH cause hypertrophy of the thecal layer which is capable of secreting large amounts of androgens. The latter presumably stimulates inhibin production, which in its turn suppresses pituitary FSH secretion. Increased secretion of inhibin by bovine granulosa cells *in vitro* by the addition of androgens has also been demonstrated by Franchimont *et al.*[52].

It therefore appears possible that inhibin acts throughout the reproductive cycle as a second negative feedback regulator in that it prevents an inappropriately high FSH secretion, and maintains a balance of the secretion of FSH and LH.

It is of particular interest that inhibin may have a direct intraovarian effect, in that chronic treatment of immature rats with hFF-inhibin and hMG brought about follicular atresia and high androgen to estrogen ratio. Whether the latter is the cause or the result of atresia is not yet known. In any event, the inhibition of aromatizing activity is apparent. It has also been shown in a different experiment that the ovulatory response to hCG (in terms of P secretion) can also be blocked by hFF-inhibin. In view of these observations it is tempting to speculate that inhibin acts primarily to regulate, through direct action processes within the gonad, and that the feedback control of gonadotropin secretion is a secondary, incidental function.

As the effect of OMI is reversible, the question arises as to why and by what means it participates in retarding the maturation of the oocyte almost to the point of ovulation. Similarly, *in vitro* studies with the luteinization inhibitor indicate its importance for the regulation of granulosa cell luteinization *in vivo* – an important event in determining the fate of a follicle. Selection of a dominant follicle depends not only on the level of FSH but also on the sensitivity of the follicle to FSH. For a given level of circulating gonadotropins the outcome, in terms of the target organ response, is the resultant of an interaction between the hormone receptor and the specific binding inhibitor. Thus, the potential significance of low molecular weight, hormone receptor-binding inhibitors capable of regulating gonadotropin action at the gonadal level is considerable.

In view of the overlap of some of the biological properties of these nonsteroidal inhibitors studied so far, the question arises whether all these factors are synthesized as independent molecules or whether they are derivatives, through the action of a specific endopeptidase, of a common precursor molecule. Further studies with chemically pure substances will be necessary to resolve this question and to determine their specific physiological roles.

Acknowledgement

We thank the National Pituitary Agency, NIADDK for providing rat FSH/ LH RIA kits. Our work was supported partly by Deutsche Forschungsgemeinschaft Grant Da 49/7 and partly by P. E. Kempkes-Stiftung, Marburg.

References

1. Richards, J. A. (1979). Hormonal control of ovarian follicular development. *Recent Prog. Horm. Res.*, **35**, 343
2. Hillier, S. G. (1981). Regulation of follicular oestrogen biosynthesis: a survey of current concepts. *J. Endocrinol.*, **89**, 3p
3. McNatty, K. P. (1981). Ovarian follicular development from the onset of luteal regression in humans and sheep. In Rolland, R., van Hall, E. P., Hillier, S. G., McNatty, K. P. and Schoemaker, J. (eds.) *Follicular Maturation and Ovulation.* pp. 1–18. (Amsterdam, Oxford, Princeton: Excerpta Medica)
4. Hillier, S. G., van Hall, E. V., van den Boogaard, A. J. M., de Zwart, F. A. and Keyzer, R. (1981). Activation and modulation of the granulosa cell aromatase system: experimental studies with rat and human ovaries. In Rolland, R., van Hall, E. V., Hillier, S. G., McNatty, K. P. and Schoemaker, J. (eds.) *Follicular Maturation and Ovulation.* pp. 51–70. (Amsterdam, Oxford, Princeton: Excerpta Medica)
5. Ross, G. T. and Hillier, S. G. (1979). Experimental aspects of follicular maturation. *Eur. J. Obstet. Gynecol. Reprod. Biol.*, **9** (3), 169
6. Hillier, S. G., Agnes, M. J., van den Boogaard, A. J. M., Reichert, L. E. Jr. and van Hall, E. V. (1980). Alterations in granulosa cell aromatase activity accompanying preovulatory follicular development in the rat ovary with evidence that 5α-reduced C_{19} steroids inhibit the aromatase reaction *in vitro. J. Endocrinol.*, **84**, 409
7. Ryan, R. G. (1981). Follicular atresia: some speculations on biochemical markers and mechanisms. In Schwartz, N. B. and Hunzicker-Dunn, M. (eds.) *Dynamics of Ovarian Function.* pp. 1–11. (New York: Raven Press)
8. Van Look, P. F. A. and Baird, D. T. (1980). Regulatory mechanisms during the menstrual cycle. *Eur. J. Obstet. Gynecol. Reprod. Biol.*, **11**, 121
9. McNatty, K. P., Moore-Smith, D., Makris, A., Osathanondh, R. and Ryan, K. (1979). The microenvironment of the human antral follicle: interrelationships among the steroidal levels in the antral fluid, the population of granulosa cells and the status of the oocytes *in vivo* and *in vitro. J. Clin. Endocrinol. Metab.*, **49**, 851
10. Channing, C. P., Hoover, D. J., Anderson, L. D. and Tanabe, K. (1982). In Fujii, T. and Channing, C. P. (eds.) *Non-steroidal Regulators in Reproductive Biology and Medicine.* pp. 41–59. (Oxford and New York: Pergamon Press)
11. Bomsel-Helmreich, O. (1983). The preovulatory human oocyte and its microenvironment. In Beier, H. M. and Lindner, H. R. (eds.) *Fertilisation of the Human Egg in vitro.* pp. 19–34. (Berlin, Heidelberg, New York, Tokyo: Springer-Verlag)
12. Zeleznik, A. J. (1981). Factors governing the selection of the preovulatory follicle in the rhesus monkey. In Rolland, R., van Hall, E. V., Hillier, S. G., McNatty, K. P. and Schoemaker, J. (eds.) *Follicular Maturation and Ovulation.* pp. 37–50. (Amsterdam, Oxford, Princeton: Excerpta Medica)
13. Hsueh, A. J. W. and Jones, P. B. C. (1981). Direct hormonal modulation of ovarian granulosa cell maturation: effect of gonadotrophin releasing hormone. In Rolland, R., van Hall, E. V., Hillier, S. G., McNatty, K. P. and Schoemaker, J. (eds.) *Follicular Maturation and Ovulation.* pp. 19–33. (Amsterdam, Oxford, Princeton: Excerpta Medica)
14. Moore, C. R. and Price, D. (1932). Gonad hormone functions, and the reciprocal influence between gonads and hypophysis with its bearing on the problem of sex hormone antagonism. *Am. J. Anat.*, **50**, 13
15. Hohlweg, W. and Junkmann, K. (1932). Die hormonal-nervöse Regulierung der Funktion des Hypophysenvorderlappens. *Klin. Wochenschr.*, **11**, 321
16. Hohlweg, W. (1934). Veränderungen des Hypophysenvorderlappens und des Ovariums nach Behandlung mit großen Dosen von Follikelhormon. *Klin. Wochenschr.*, **13**, 92
17. De Jong, F. H. (1979). Inhibin – fact or artefact. *Mol. Cell. Endocrinol.*, **13**, 1
18. Channing, C. P., Anderson, L. D., Hoover, D. J., Kolena, J., Osteen, K. G., Pomerantz, S. H. and Tanabe, K. (1982). The role of nonsteroidal regulators in control of oocyte and follicular maturation. *Recent Prog. Horm. Res.*, **38**, 331
19. Grady, R. R., Charlesworth, M. C. and Schwartz, N. B. (1982). Characterization of the FSH suppressing activity in follicular fluid. *Recent Prog. Horm. Res.*, **38**, 409

20. Chari, S., Hopkinson, C. R. N., Daume, E. and Sturm, G. (1979). Purification of inhibin from human follicular fluid. *Acta Endocrinol.*, **90**, 157
21. Chari, S., Duraiswami, S., Daume, E. and Sturm, G. (1981). Biological characteristics of inhibin from human ovarian follicular fluid. In Semm, K. and Mettler, L. (eds.) *Human Reproduction*. pp. 463–467. (Amsterdam, Oxford, Princeton: Excerpta Medica)
22. Chari, S., Duraiswami, S., Daume, E. and Sturm, G. (1982). Physicochemical and biological characteristics of human ovarian follicular fluid inhibin. In Fujii, T. and Channing, C. P. (eds.) *Non-steroidal Regulators in Reproductive Biology and Medicine*. pp. 61–72. (Oxford and New York: Pergamon Press)
23. Daume, E., Chari, S., Sturm, G., Hillensjoe, T. and Magnusson, C. (1981). Non-steroidal ovarian inhibitors in human follicular fluid. In Rolland, R., van Hall, E. V., Hillier, S. G., McNatty, K. P. and Schoemaker, J. (eds.) *Follicular Maturation and Ovulation*. pp. 237–248. (Amsterdam, Oxford, Princeton: Excerpta Medica)
24. Kraulis, A., Traikov, H., Sharpe, M., Ruf, K. B. and Naftolin, F. (1978). Steroid induction of gonadotrophin surges in the immature rat. I. Priming effects of androgens. *Endocrinology*, **103**, 1822
25. Kraulis, A., Traikov, H., Ruf, K. B. and Naftolin, F. (1978). Steroid induction of gonadotrophin surges in immature rat. II. Triggering ability of progesterone metabolites, adrenocortical hormones and adrenocorticotropin. *Endocrinology*, **103**, 1829
26. Hopkinson, C. R. N., Chari, S., Sturm, G. and Hirschhäuser, C. (1979). Study of testicular feedback in male rats using artificial cryptorchidism as a model. *Horm. Res.*, **10**, 310
27. Bronson, F. H. and Channing, C. P. (1978). Suppression of serum follicle-stimulating hormone by follicular fluid in the maximally estrogenized, ovariectomized mouse. *Endocrinology*, **103**, 1895
28. Chari, S., Aumüller, G., Daume, E., Sturm, G. and Hopkinson, C. R. N. (1981). The effects of human follicular fluid inhibin on the morphology of the ovary of the immature rat. *Arch. Gynecol.*, **230**, 239
29. Condon, T. P., Leipheimer, R. and Curry, J. J. (1983). Preliminary evidence for a CNS site of action for ovarian inhibin. *Life Sci.*, **32**, 1691
30. DiZerega, G. S., Goebelsmann, U. and Nakamura, R. M. (1982). Identification protein(s) secreted by the preovulatory ovary which suppresses the follicle response to gonadotropins. *J. Clin. Endocrinol. Metab.*, **54**, 1091
31. Peluso, J. J., Stude, D. and Steger, R. W. (1980). Role of androgens in hCG-induced ovulation in PMSG-primed immature rats. *Acta Endocrinol.*, **93**, 505
32. Hillensjoe, T., Chari, S., Magnusson, C., Daume, E. and Sturm, G. (1981). Inhibitory effects of low molecular weight fractions of human follicular fluid upon rat granulosa cells and oocytes *in vitro*. In Semm, K. and Mettler, L. (eds.) *Human Reproduction*. pp. 458–462. (Amsterdam, Oxford, Princeton: Excerpta Medica)
33. Hillensjoe, T., Chari, S., Nilsson, L., Hamburger, L., Daume, E. and Sturm, G. (1983). Inhibition of progesterone in cultured human granulosa cells by a low molecular weight fraction of follicular fluid. *J. Clin. Endocrinol. Metab.*, **56**, 835
34. Tsafriri, A., Pomerantz, S. H. and Channing, C. P. (1976). Inhibition of oocyte maturation by porcine follicular fluid: partial characterization of the inhibitor. *Biol. Reprod.*, **14**, 511
35. Stone, S. L., Pomerantz, S. H., Schwartz-Kripner, A. and Channing, C. P. (1978). Inhibitor of oocyte maturation from porcine follicular fluid: further purification and evidence for reversible action. *Biol. Reprod.*, **19**, 585
36. Pomerantz, S. H., Channing, C. P. and Tsafriri, A. (1979). Studies on the purification and action of an oocyte maturation inhibitor isolated from porcine follicular fluid. In Gross, E. and Meienhofer, J. (eds.) *Peptides: Structure and Biological Function*. pp. 765–774. (Pierce Chemical Co.)
37. Hillensjoe, T., Pomerantz, S. H., Kripner, A. S., Anderson, L. D. and Channing, C. P. (1980). Inhibition of cumulus cell progesterone secretion by low molecular weight fractions of porcine follicular fluid which also inhibit oocyte maturation. *Endocrinology*, **106**, 584
38. Tsafriri, A., Channing, C. P., Pomerantz, S. H. and Lindner, H. R. (1977). Inhibition of maturation of isolated rat oocytes by porcine follicular fluid. *J. Endocrinol.*, **75**, 285
39. Hillensjoe, T., Batta, S. K., Kripner, A. S., Wentz, A. C., Sulewski, J. and Channing, C. P. (1978). Inhibitory effect of human follicular fluid upon maturation of porcine oocytes in culture. *J. Clin. Endocrinol. Metab.*, **47**, 1332

40. Chari, S., Hillensjoe, T., Magnusson, C., Sturm, G. and Daume, E. (1983). *In vitro* inhibition of rat oocyte meiosis by human follicular fluid fractions. *Arch. Gynecol.*, **233**, 155

41. Darga, N. C. and Reichert, L. E. Jr. (1978). Some properties of the interaction of follicle stimulating hormone with bovine granulosa cells and its inhibition by follicular fluid. *Biol. Reprod.*, **19**, 235

42. Daume, E., Chari, S., Hopkinson, C. R. N. and Sturm, G. (1979). Inhibition of follicle stimulating hormone binding to granulosa cells *in vitro* by human follicular fluid. *Arch. Gynecol.*, **227**, 289

43. Daume, E., Chari, S. and Sturm, G. (1981). Follicle-stimulating hormone binding inhibitor (FSH-BI) in human follicular fluid. In Semm, K. and Mettler, L. (eds.) *Human Reproduction*. pp. 468–471. (Amsterdam, Oxford, Princeton: Excerpta Medica)

44. Reichert, L. E. Jr., Sanzo, M. A. and Darga, N. A. (1979). Studies on a low molecular weight follicle-stimulating hormone binding inhibitor from human serum. *J. Clin. Endocrinol. Metab.*, **49**, 866

45. Ledwitz-Rigby, F. and Rigby, B. W. (1981). Ovarian inhibitors and stimulators of granulosa cell maturation and luteinisation. In Franchimont, P. and Channing, C. P. (eds.) *Intragonadal Regulation of Reproduction*. pp. 97–131. (London, New York, Toronto, Sydney, San-Francisco: Academic Press)

46. DiZerega, G. S., Turner, C. K., Stouffer, R. L., Anderson, L. D., Channing, C. P. and Hodgen, G. D. (1981). Suppression of follicle-stimulating hormone dependent folliculogenesis during the primate ovarian cycle. *J. Clin. Endocrinol. Metab.*, **52**, 451

47. Ross, G. T., Cargille, C. M., Lipsett, M. B., Rayford, P. L., Marshall, J. R., Strott, C. A. and Rodbard, D. (1970). Pituitary and gonadal induced ovulatory cycles. *Recent Prog. Horm. Res.*, **26**, 1

48. Wilks, J. W., Hodgen, G. D. and Ross, G. T. (1976). Luteal phase defects in the rhesus monkey: the significance of serum FSH:LH ratios. *J. Clin. Endocrinol. Metab.*, **43**, 1261

49. Rebar, R., Judd, H. L., Yen, S. S. C., Rakoff, J., Vandenberg, G. and Naftolin, F. (1976). Characterization of the inappropriate gonadotrophin secretion in polycystic ovary syndrome. *J. Clin. Invest.*, **57**, 1320

50. Yen, S. S. C., Vela, P. and Rankin, J. (1970). Inappropriate secretion of follicle-stimulating hormone and luteinizing hormone in polycycstic ovarian disease. *J. Clin. Endocrinol. Metab.*, **30**, 435

51. Tanabe, K., Gagliano, P., Channing, C. P., Nakamura, Y., Yoshimura, I., Iizuka, R., Fortuny, A., Sulewski, J. and Rezai, N. (1983). Levels of inhibin-F activity and steroids in human follicular fluid from normal women with polycystic ovarian disease. *J. Clin. Endocrinol. Metab.*, **57**, 24

52. Franchimont, P., Verstraelen-Proyard, J., Hazee-Hagelstein, M. T., Renard, Ch., Demoulin, A., Bourguignon, J. P. and Hustin, J. (1979). Inhibin: from concept to reality. *Vit. Horm.*, **37**, 243

Discussion

Runnebaum	You have shown quite different sites of action of big inhibin. What is the main effect of big inhibin? Is it dependent on the concentration, and is there any indication for specific binding sites in the hypothalamus?
Daume	At the moment we do not know much about the physiological role and the mechanism of action of inhibin-like substances. We are still at work to isolate and characterize the active fractions and to develop a sensitive test-system for inhibin. The results of our *in vivo* experiments indicate that inhibin acts mainly as a local factor at the ovarian level. So far, we have no data on specific binding-sites for inhibin.
Bettendorf	In your *in vitro* experiments you used doses up to 150 μg. How pure was the material you used, can you exclude an unspecific effect of some other protein, and what is the concentration of inhibin in the follicular fluid?
Daume	Utilizing isoelectric focusing and gel electrophoresis, big inhibin was found to be homogeneous, while we were not able as yet to isolate small inhibin. We succeeded in enriching the biological activity by a factor of 100. Moreover, we have demonstrated that albumin and other serum proteins do not exert any inhibin-like effect, although big inhibin has a structure similar to that of albumin. This is, however, the reason for the cross-reaction of albumin with antibodies which had been raised against inhibin. Therefore, we have not been able to measure the inhibin concentration in the follicular fluid.
Rothchild	It is almost impossible to explain the course of follicular development by the effects of gonadotropins alone. There have to be intrafollicular regulation mechanisms, probably of an inhibitory nature, because normal follicular development is not the result of an uncontrolled stimulation. As it was shown that the granulosa cells and the oocyte are very rich in prolactin, it was speculated that inhibin, OMI and some other substances in the follicular fluid may be breakdown products of prolactin.
Koninckx	You have investigated the effect of inhibin upon the oocyte and the granulosa cells; but I wonder why you did not look at the stromal sites of the ovary, although you have observed that the testosterone secretion was increased. In our own laboratory another ovarian factor is under investigation which is secreted by the granulosa cells and specifically induces androgen secretion.
Kuhl	Have you investigated the possibility whether big inhibin is a pre- or prohormone of small inhibin or of other peptides? In this way, the effect of big inhibin upon the hypothalamus, e.g., might be a secondary one.
Daume	We do not think that our big inhibin fraction (MW 23000) is a parent substance of small inhibin. There are reports on big inhibin with MW between 80000 and 160000, which possibly have both activities. At the moment it is not proven that our small inhibin fraction (MW below 1000), which also has OMI activity, is a peptide.
Wentz	Is there a difference in the follicular size that determines whether you obtain small or big inhibin?

19

Daume	This was not investigated because we are working with crude material from pools of follicular fluid and not with individual samples.
Breckwoldt	If inhibin is a peptide, there should be a breakdown of the molecule by exposing it to heat.
Daume	The big inhibin is destroyed by heat, the small inhibin is resistant.
Braendle	In one of your experiments with rats, the treatment with hMG could not overcome the action of inhibin. Did you ever use FSH in your experimental model?
Daume	We did not use pure FSH.
Dericks-Tan	Schenken and Hodgen (*J. Clin. Endocrinol. Metab.* **57** (1983), 50) showed that hyperstimulation of the ovary with FSH abolished the LH surge in monkeys, indicating the existence of a factor which specifically reduces the LH response. Did you find a fraction with LH inhibiting activity?
Daume	With our inhibin fraction we could either suppress FSH or both FSH and LH, depending upon the physiological situation. The suppression of LH, however, is inconsistent; no experiment is like the other, and we have no explanation for that.

2
Pathophysiology of the inadequate corpus luteum

I. ROTHCHILD

If the inadequate corpus luteum (ICL) is indeed one of the causes of otherwise unexplained infertility[1], knowing its cause is absolutely essential to treating and even diagnosing it. My responsibility, therefore, is a large one and rather frightening, because I do not think the commonly accepted causes are the right ones, and I can only speculate about other possibilities.

COMMONLY ACCEPTED OR SUGGESTED CAUSES OF ICL

FSH deficiency during the early follicular phase

Background

This idea has been held for a long time (for references see: Refs. 1–3). McNatty[4] thought that FSH deficiency reduced the number of follicular granulosa cells, and therefore the size of the CL, since the CL grows primarily by cellular hypertrophy. Various clinical observations, for example that vigorous aspiration of an oocyte, by removing too many granulosa cells, causes ICL formation[5], have also tended to support this idea. Depression of early follicular phase FSH levels in monkeys by treatment with female inhibin also led to ICL formation[3]. The hypothesis is reasonable since the rate of progesterone (P) secretion is directly proportional to the total mass of luteal tissue, at least in some species[6].

Evaluation of the hypothesis

All ICL are not necessarily associated with FSH deficiency and vice-versa, nor do all ICL contain fewer cells than normal. The inhibin-treated monkeys had a normal number of cells/CL, although they were smaller than normal[3]. This implies, however, that FSH deficiency is only part of a syndrome affecting CL growth. FSH treatment of the affected monkeys, in fact, only tended to raise serum P levels, but did not restore them to a normal pattern[3]. Even in the report of Garcia *et al.*[5] there was no correlation between individual cell counts and ICL formation.

Some findings do not fit well with the hypothesis. In women in whom ovulation was induced with gonadotropins, there were no differences in follicular phase estrogen levels between those who conceived and those with short luteal phases who did not[7]. There was also no difference from normal estrogen levels before and after ovulation in a group of infertile women with subnormal P levels[8]. Not all women with ICL have low estrogen levels[9]. Such observations are important, for if FSH is so deficient that granulosa cell development is affected enough to cause ICL formation, estrogen secretion should also be deficient (see below).

It is curious that in monkeys actively immunized against β-LH, ICL formation was associated with higher than normal FSH levels[10]. It is also very curious that no-one has asked why it is only FSH and not LH secretion also which is depressed. Furthermore, the association is primarily statistical, and it is usually impossible to predict, in any individual, the pattern of one hormone from that of the other. All these features of the association suggest that FSH deficiency does not cause an ICL, but that it and the ICL are the results of a common cause. For example, an abnormality of female inhibin production could depress both FSH and P secretion.

Luteal phase deficiency of LH

Background

The primitive mammal's CL was probably autonomous; later it became responsive to, and then dependent on, extrinsic factors[6]. Among many polyestrous eutheria, including primates, an increasing dependency on LH seems to have accompanied a decreasing capacity for autonomy. For example, induced CL in hypophysectomized women functioned normally only in response to LH or HCG[11], and in monkeys, treatment with an antisera to LH induced luteolysis[12]. LH (or hCG) will also increase P production by human or monkey CL cells *in vitro*; such information, however, does not prove that LH is an essential luteotropin, since it will also have this effect *in vitro* on CL which *in vivo* can secrete P in the absence of LH[6]. Other evidence also suggests an association between LH deficiency during the luteal phase and ICL formations[2, 3, 10, 13–15].

Evaluation of the hypothesis

Unlike other endocrine glands, in which the level of activity is determined by the circulating level of the tropic hormone, the CL secretes P in no obvious relation to the circulating level of its presumptive luteotropin[6]. In the human, in fact, the P and LH levels are inversely related to each other. LH, therefore, must permit the CL to secrete P, but it does not specifically determine how much it secretes. The important question thus is: How little is *too* little? Gaps and unresolved discrepancies in our knowledge make it impossible to answer this question now; nevertheless, some interesting possibilities exist.

In the case of the human, we know a little about the effects of chronic hypophysectomy on CL induced by gonadotropin treatment[11] and nothing about how acute hypophysectomy would affect a naturally formed CL. In one study of monkeys, both complete and sham hypophysectomy induced luteolysis[16], but Asch et al.[17] recently found that neither acute nor chronic hypophysectomy seriously affects the activity of naturally formed or induced CL, respectively. Not all eutherian CL have lost the capacity for autonomy[6], and the primate CL may really be among those with an appreciable capacity for autonomy.

The rat's CL become so dependent on LH during the second week after ovulation that a single injection of an antiserum to LH induces luteolysis very quickly[6]. In monkeys, however, a single LH antiserum injection induces only a temporary fall in the P level, and several repeated injections are needed to induce luteolysis[12].

Thus, the evidence that LH is an *essential* luteotropin in primates is not as definite as it once was, and we should ask whether an ICL is more often the result of a defect in response than of too little stimulation. That the ICL sometimes responds to hCG does not make the question inappropriate, since hCG can affect the CL when LH cannot[18]. In any case, a CL which responds normally to hCG may not really be inadequate.

In the monkeys actively immunized against β-LH[10] some findings raise questions about whether ICL formation is just an effect of too little LH. These monkeys are able to ovulate. Does this mean that LH bound to antibody can induce ovulation but cannot support luteal P secretion? Or was there enough free LH in the circulation for ovulation but not for the CL? The improbability of either possibility suggests an intrinsic luteal defect.

Nevertheless, one cannot altogether dismiss the possibility that too little LH may sometimes make a CL inadequate. The deficiency, however, may be expressed subtly, perhaps, as with LH dependency in rats, in connection with a sudden increase in the CL's need for LH at a critical stage of its life. The deficiency may also not be apparent from the RIA-determined serum LH level, since this is not always equivalent to the level of bioactive LH[19].

Hyperprolactinaemia as a cause of ICL

Background

When PRL RIAs became available, the association between galactorrhea and anovulation proved to be in most cases (as one might expect) an association between hyperprolactinaemia and anovulation. A similar association between hyperprolactinaemia and ICL formation was also suspected. For example, induced hyperprolactinaemia in women is frequently accompanied by ICL formation[20, 21] and treatment of hyperprolactinaemic women with 2-Br-α-ergocryptine improves their CL activity[22]. It is generally believed that too much PRL may cause ICL formation by interfering directly either with follicle development or with the CL's ability to secrete P. I will try to analyse each of these ideas.

23

Evaluation of the hypothesis

PRL and follicle development. PRL treatment of intact rats depresses follicular production of estrogens *in vitro*[23]. PRL in the medium also depresses aromatase activity of rat granulosa cells *in vitro*[24, 25], and of androgen production *in vitro* by rat theca cells[25]. In women, if the level of circulating PRL is consistently above 100 ng/ml, PRL in follicular fluid is above 20 ng/ml, and the follicles have fewer granulosa cells and make less estrogen than normal[26].

Such information implies that PRL inhibits the *proper* development of the follicle, but this may not be true. The oocyte and granulosa cells normally are especially rich in PRL and its receptors[2, 27, 28]. The PRL molecule may be the source of special inhibitory substances in follicular fluid[27], which may be necessary for normal follicular development, since this is the result of *controlled* stimulation; PRL's interaction with prostaglandins in the control of cell membrane fluidity[29] is probably also an important aspect of normal development. Other things than the PRL level itself may determine its concentration and effects within the follicle. At circulating PRL levels below 100 ng/ml, for example, its level in follicular fluid remained at about 20 ng/ml, regardless of the circulating level or the condition of the follicles[26]; at higher levels the defects in follicle development were probably the result of the accompanying abnormalities of gonadotropin secretion[30] (see below).

The *in vitro* data in rats are at odds with the lack of effect of PRL on the rat ovary's response to gonadotropins *in vivo*[31], the lack of effect of hyperprolactinaemia in normogonadotropic monkeys on the ovarian hormone patterns of the ovulation cycle[32], the stimulation by gonadotropins of PRL receptors in granulosa cells[33] (which may be part of the reason why PRL facilitates puberty), and with the absence of any inhibiting effect of PRL on follicle activity *in vitro* in other species, as e.g., the cow[34].

PRL and CL function. An inverse relationship between PRL in the medium and P produced by human CL cells *in vitro*[35] is the main source of the idea that too much PRL is bad for the human CL. Actually, however, PRL has luteotropic effects in primates[6, 32, 36–38] and although it is not an essential luteotropin, it is also unlikely that it depresses P production.

Very high serum PRL levels occur as frequently in women during the cycle of conception as in women with short luteal phases who do not conceive[39]. Spontaneous high PRL levels[40, 41] and even induced hyperprolactinaemia[42] do not affect luteal P secretion during early human pregnancy. Tan and Biggs[43], using human CL, and Stouffer *et al.*[36] using monkey CL, found that PRL does not inhibit P production *in vitro*. In hyperprolactinaemic monkeys, luteal phase P levels are indistinguishable from normal except for a slower rate of regression in the former[32].

Conclusions. The defects of follicle development associated with hyperprolactinaemia do not seem to be direct effects of PRL, nor does PRL seem to affect the CL directly. The association between hyperprolactinaemia and ICL formation, therefore, most likely arises from the disordered gonadotropin secretion[30] which so frequently accompanies hyperprolactinaemia.

OTHER THEORETICALLY POSSIBLE CAUSES OF ICL FORMATION

The association between certain kinds of anovulation and ICL formation

Background

A few conditions exist in which ICL formation seems to occur consistently, and comparatively frequently. These are anovulatory conditions in which the potential for ovulation remains intact; ovulation, therefore, can occur, but infrequently and irregularly. I will first mention a few of the main features of this association (which is not peculiar to people) and then try to analyse its cause.

Postmenarche and premenopause in humans. These conditions are typified by both irregularities of menstruation, a result of anovulation, and a high incidence of short luteal phases[44]. A similar high frequency of ICL formation occurs during puberty in monkeys[45].

Seasonal anovulation in monkeys. During the summer, monkeys tend to become amenorrhoeic or irregularly menstrual, the results of anovulation. The incidence of ICL formation also rises at this time[46].

Seasonal anestrus in sheep, and related conditions in pigs, goats, and cattle. Gonadotropins are secreted and follicles grow during this period of anovulation in sheep but somewhat differently from the breeding season pattern[47]. Ovulation can be induced, but the circulating P level is abnormally low, although the length of the luteal phase is normal[48]. The abnormality is not due to the seasonal hyperprolactinaemia[49]. The association between anovulation and ICL formation also appears in the smaller than normal incidence of induced ovulations[49]. During the summer pigs tend to be anovulatory or to form ICL[50]. In *goats*, short luteal phases occur more frequently early in, than at the height of, the breeding season[51]. *Brahman cattle* tend to form ICL during their seasonal anestrus[52].

The puerperium, lactation and hyperprolactinaemia. Even in non-lactating normoprolactinaemic women, the transition from pregnancy to regular ovulation cycles is associated with evidence of ICL formation[53]. In late lactation, when PRL levels are virtually normal, anovulatory cycles and ICL formation increase in frequency[54]. Similarly, among cattle, short luteal phases occur frequently after the first ovulation postpartum[55, 56].

Possible causes of the association

In these forms of anovulation gonadotropin secretion is subnormal[21, 47, 57, 58], usually because of decreases in rate and/or amplitude of the secretion pulses. The hormones' effectiveness can also decrease because of either a change in metabolism or in the properties of the secreted hormone itself. Differences from normal in CNS activity cause these abnormalities; they can also be maintained or aggravated by the feedback effects of the abnormal ovarian hormones they induce. They are the most important cause of ICL formation.

Ovulation and formation of an adequate CL depend essentially on the kind of LH surge the preovulatory follicle induces, and on how it responds to it. The response must be intimately related to follicle growth, i.e. to estrogen secretion. The granulosa cells make estrogens in response to FSH, which stimulates their aromatase activity. The theca cells, in response to LH, make the androgen precursors. Follicles grow exponentially because estrogens stimulate their own production, through their effects on their own and FSH receptors in granulosa cells, and because they are the main stimulus of granulosa cell proliferation[59]. With FSH they also eventually induce LH receptors in the granulosa cells[59].

It would be difficult to exaggerate the importance of androgens, and so of LH, in these interdependencies. Besides serving as estrogen precursors[60], androgens synergize with FSH equally well in stimulating aromatase activity in, and P production by, the granulosa cells[61]. They are probably essential for ovulation[62], an effect possibly related to how they induce atresia (see below). The role of P in these relationships is still unclear. However, if estrogens can indeed inhibit thecal androgen production[60] *in vivo*, this action must be counterbalanced in some way, for otherwise the follicle would not grow; granulosa cell P may have this effect, perhaps by serving as an androgen precursor.

The self-stimulating quality of estrogen production may buffer the follicle against large fluctuations in FSH secretion, but no such process protects androgen production. Even minor fluctuations of LH secretion, therefore, can have serious effects, e.g. an androgen deficiency, which by reducing estrogen production below an optimum, may induce atresia indirectly, or an androgen excess, which will do so directly. Almost all the follicles of a cohort undergo atresia because of how easily this balance is upset. It is interesting that abnormalities of LH, rather than of FSH, secretion also seem to be typical of the anovulations of puberty, etc. The nocturnal surge of LH in human puberty[58], the selective depression of LH during lactation[57] or in hypothalamically lesioned monkeys treated with slow GnRH pulses[63] and the seasonal anestrus in sheep[47] are only a few examples of this.

The rare follicle which escapes atresia under normal conditions is the one which maintains a steady increase in its capacity for estrogen production. On the even more rare occasions when a follicle reaches the stage of preovulation in these anovulations, its fate as a normal CL is still not assured, for it must still induce an LH surge as well as respond to it. Since this depends on the pituitary's response to GnRH, the stimulation of this response by estrogen, and on the rate and probably amplitude of the GnRH secretion pulses, the LH surge may not always be normal. The combination of a potentially abnormal response of the follicle to an LH surge which may also deviate from normal is almost certainly the most important reason for the frequency of ICL formation in these anovulations.

Atresia, induced in preovulatory rat follicles by barbiturate-induced delay of the LH surge[64], is accompanied, as in normal ovulation, by a fall in estrogen and androgen secretion, and by a rise in P secretion (due to thecal luteinization), the duration and rate of which resemble that of a human ICL. Not only, therefore, is there no sharp distinction between atresia and luteinization, but one may even think of luteinization as a form of atresia. Androgens may be required for ovulation[62], possibly because their effects resemble the atresia they induce in younger than preovulatory follicles. A deficiency of androgen production, secondary to one of LH, therefore, could be among the more important reasons that the outcome of the exchange between follicle and LH surge is often an ICL.

Thus, under these conditions, the follicle may help drive itself into paths that normal conditions keep closed. It may neither ovulate nor luteinize; it may ovulate but luteinize poorly or not at all; it may luteinize poorly or completely without ovulating[65]; and, of course, it may even ovulate and luteinize completely. Which of these fates overtakes it may depend not only on the general relationships discussed so far, but on an unknown number of those to be considered in the next section.

Causes arising from defects in certain aspects of CL function

The causes described so far are primarily extrinsic ones, although some, of course, can induce intrinsic defects in the CL through their actions on the follicle. The orientation now will be primarily, but not exclusively, on intrinsic defects.

Autonomy

I have already mentioned that the primate CL may be more autonomous than was supposed[17]. The gonadotropins probably induce the capacity for autonomy in the follicular granulosa cells. One of the effects of the conditions of anovulation may be to reduce this capacity, thus making the CL abnormally dependent on LH. This may be why a more than adequate LH level for a normal CL is an LH deficiency for an ICL.

Prostaglandins (PGs)

Evidence that certain PGs cause luteolysis in primates[6] continues to accumulate[66-69], and it is unrealistic to ignore the importance of PGs in controlling the human CL. One way an ICL may arise, therefore, is through disruption of the normal relationships between P and PG production within the CL, possibly because of abnormal gonadotropin secretion.

Estrogens

Whether estrogens induce luteolysis in primates[6] directly, or by depressing LH secretion, is uncertain. In two recent studies the authors favoured the latter explanation, but they failed to test it by seeing whether LH would prevent the luteolytic effect of estrogens[70, 71]. The estrogens' luteolytic effect, like that of PGs[6], is proportional to the age of the CL[72]. Other evidence also suggests a relation to intraluteal PG[6], including the finding that suppressing PRL secretion in women[37] or baboons[38] increases the luteolytic effect of estrogens. PRL may suppress PG production under some conditions[6] (Ueda, Ochiai and Rothchild, in preparation). An abnormality of luteal estrogen production, therefore, may reduce the CL's secretion.

Female inhibin

Follicular fluid and a variety of non-steroidal substances secreted into it are products of granulosa cell activity; some of these, at least, are due to FSH stimulation. As far as the ICL is concerned, female inhibin is probably the most interesting. In the cow, for example, the production of P by follicular granulosa cells is inversely related to their production of inhibin and inhibin production is, at least in part, stimulated by androgens[73]. It would be reasonable to suppose that P production by follicular granulosa cells is directly related to that of luteinized granulosa cells. Androgens, in synergism with FSH, also stimulate granulosa cell P production[61]. A derangement which diverts the androgen effect from P to inhibin production would thus reduce the cells' potential capacity for P production. If inhibin secretion also persisted after luteinization (the normal CL does not make inhibin)[73] this would also reduce P secretion.

Oxytocin and relaxin

Although neither oxytocin nor relaxin seem to be luteolytic, or even necessary for P production, research into their roles in regulating CL activity is fairly new, and a disturbed relation between them and P production cannot be eliminated as a cause of ICL formation.

A luteolytic effect of LH

Under some circumstances the luteolytic actions of LH may outweigh its luteotropic ones. For example, GnRH analogues, although they induce luteolysis in primates in vivo, do not do so in vitro[43]. In rats, however, these compounds are directly luteolytic. The luteolytic effects of GnRH in primates, therefore, may be due to increased LH secretion.

LH may induce luteolysis acutely by desensitization, or chronically by facilitating intraluteal PG production. Both effects imply that something else potentiates them.

28

The formation of ICL through the effects of ICL

P is important in maintaining the regularity of ovulation cycles, probably, among other reasons, because of its ability to potentiate pituitary gonado-tropin secretion, especially LH[74]. It is, therefore, not too far-fetched to suppose that the accidental formation of an ICL may lead to the formation of another ICL in the next cycle, and so on. How much this accounts for most ICLs is, of course, unknown; but the high incidence of cures claimed for the effects of P treatment suggest that it can be significant. The sporadic nature of ICL formation in general, however, suggests that some process prevents it from being permanently self-perpetuating.

Still other possibilities

Defects associated with the reorganization of the cytoskeleton during lutein-ization, with the CL's use of circulating lipoproteins as the main source of cholesterol for P synthesis, with how its hormone receptors are internalized and metabolized, with how its blood flow is regulated, etc., may be involved in any of the above-mentioned causes, or may be causes in their own right.

CONDITIONS UNDER WHICH ICL FORMATION MAY BE ILLUSORY

Changes in the metabolic clearance rate (MCR) of P

We judge the inadequacy of the human CL on the basis of assumptions that have not always (or never?) been tested. We do not measure the secretion rate of P, but assume that its circulating level is always a direct measure of how much P is being secreted. It is true that the MCR of P in people does not change in a large variety of conditions[75], but this does not mean that it will not change in *all* conditions. In sheep, for example, the rate of P secretion also usually parallels P's circulating level but during the seasonal anestrus the MCR of P rises[48]. What appears to be ICL induced during anestrus, there-fore, may really be normal CL. Obviously, if in some cases of suspected ICL, it turns out that the MCR of P has increased, the problem is not in the CL but in how P is metabolized.

The CL's response to hCG

The question of how adequate a CL is in terms of its response to hCG has only rarely been asked[13], but the question is of first importance. It does not take very much P to induce normal secretory changes in the endometrium[76] and P can fall to very low levels for several days early in pregnancy without inducing abortion[38]. The adequacy of a CL, therefore, is not always synony-mous with the amount of P it secretes at a given moment; more important is its potential ability, and as far as infertility is concerned, this means how well it responds to the hormonal changes that follow implantation. Their ability to delay the regression phase of P secretion is more important than the ability of hCG to raise the rate of P secretion[18], but the latter can be a measure of the former. Such a specific test of CL adequacy, in suspected cases of ICL, has never been consistently applied, but it would be the most significant of all, since it should distinguish between CL which are truly inadequate and those which only appear to be so.

SUMMARY AND CONCLUSIONS

There is little justification for considering a follicular phase deficiency of FSH, or a luteal phase deficiency of LH, as important causes of inadequate CL (ICL) formation, although one cannot eliminate them completely. Hyperprolactinaemia itself does not seem to affect either the follicle or the CL adversely, and the association with ICL formation is probably the result of disordered gonadotropin secretion. The richest source of information about what causes ICL is the association between ICL formation and the anovulations typical of adolescence, the puerperium, lactation, and hyper-prolactinaemia in people and in monkeys, cows, sheep, goats and pigs, and of the seasonal anestrus in the latter animals. The common factor may be a lower than normal level of LH secretion and/or bioactivity, which results in changes in follicle growth and luteinization that reduce the CL's capacity for P production. Other possible causes, separate from or part of these, could include: a reduced capacity for autonomous P production; disorders of production of PGs, estrogens, female inhibin, oxytocin or relaxin; an exaggerated luteolytic effect of LH; and even that an ICL may induce ICL formation. ICL formation may also sometimes be illusory, e.g. if the MCR of P has increased, or if the CL's response to hCG is normal.

References

1. Wentz, A. C. (1982). Diagnosing luteal phase inadequacy. *Fertil. Steril.*, **37**, 334
2. Andrews, W. C. (1979). Luteal phase defects. *Fertil. Steril.*, **32**, 501
3. DiZerga, G. and Hodgen, G. D. (1981). Luteal phase dysfunction infertility: a sequel to aberrant folliculogenesis. *Fertil. Steril.*, **35**, 489
4. McNatty, K. P. (1979). Follicular determinants of corpus luteum function in the human ovary. In Channing, C. P. *et al.* (eds.) *Ovarian Follicle and Corpus Luteum Function.* p. 465. (New York: Plenum Press)
5. Garcia, J., Jones, G. S., Acosta, A. A. and Wright, G. L. Jr. (1981). Corpus luteum function after follicle aspiration for oocyte retrieval. *Fertil. Steril.*, **36**, 565
6. Rothchild, I. (1981). The regulation of the mammalian corpus luteum. *Recent Prog. Horm. Res.*, **37**, 183
7. Olson, J. L., Rebar, R. W., Schreiber, J. R. and Vaitukaitis, J. L. (1983). Shortened luteal phase after ovulation induction with human menopausal gonadotropin and human chorionic gonadotropin. *Fertil. Steril.*, **39**, 284
8. Driessen, F., Kremer, J., Alsbach, G. P. J. and Kroon, R. A. (1980). Serum progesterone and oestradiol concentrations in women with unexplained infertility. *Br. J. Obstet. Gynaecol.*, **87**, 619

9. Goldstein, D., Zuckerman, H., Harpaz, S., Barkai, J., Geva, A., Gordon, S., Shalev, E. and Schwartz, M. (1982). Correlation between estradiol and progesterone in cycles with luteal phase deficiency. *Fertil. Steril.*, **37**, 348

10. Thau, R. B., Yamamoto, Y., Sundaram, K. and Spinola, P. G. (1983). Human chorionic gonadotropin stimulates luteal function in rhesus monkeys immunized against the beta-subunit of ovine luteinizing hormone. *Endocrinology*, **112**, 277

11. Vande Wiele, R. L. *et al.* (1970). Mechanisms regulating the menstrual cycle in women. *Recent Prog. Horm. Res.*, **26**, 63

12. Moudgal, N. R., Macdonald, G. J. and Greep, R. D. (1972). Role of endogenous primate LH in maintaining corpus luteum function of the monkey. *J. Clin. Endocrinol. Metab.*, **35**, 113

13. Jones, G. S., Aksel, S. and Wentz, A. C. (1974). Serum progesterone values in the luteal phase defects. Effect of chorionic gonadotropin. *Obstet. Gynecol.*, **44**, 26

14. Wilks, J. W., Hodgen, G. D. and Ross, G. T. (1976). Luteal phase defects in the rhesus monkey: the significance of serum FSH:LH ratios. *J. Clin. Endocrinol. Metab.*, **43**, 1261

15. Sakai, C. N. and Channing, C. P. (1979). Evidence for alterations in luteinizing hormone secreted in rhesus monkeys with normal and inadequate luteal phases using radioreceptor and radioimmunoassay. *Endocrinology*, **104**, 1217

16. Knobil, E., Neill, J. D. and Johansson, E. D. B. (1968). Influence of hypophysectomy, sham hypophysectomy and other surgical procedures on luteal function in the rhesus monkey. *Endocrinology*, **82**, 410

17. Asch, R. H., Abou-Samra, M., Braunstein, G. D. and Pauerstein, C. J. (1982). Luteal function in hypophysectomized rhesus monkeys. *J. Clin. Endocrinol. Metab.*, **55**, 154

18. Rothchild, I. (1982). Effect of pregnancy on the corpus luteum. In van der Molen, H. J. *et al.* (eds.) *Hormonal Factors in Fertility, Infertility and Contraception.* pp. 51–72. (Amsterdam: Elsevier)

19. Dufau, M. L., Hodgen, G. D., Goodman, A. L. and Catt, K. J. (1977). Bioassay of circulating luteinizing hormone in rhesus monkey: comparison with radioimmunoassay during physiological changes. *Endocrinology*, **100**, 1557

20. L'Hermite, M., Michaux-Duchene, A. and Robyn, C. (1979). Tiapride-induced chronic hyperprolactinaemia: interference with the human menstrual cycle. *Acta Endocrinol.* (Copenhagen), **92**, 214

21. Kauppila, A., Leinonen, P. and Ylostalo, P. (1982). Metoclopramide-induced hyperprolactinaemia impairs ovarian follicle maturation and corpus luteum function in women. *J. Clin. Endocrinol. Metab.*, **54**, 955

22. Bohnet, H. G., Hanker, J. P., Horowski, R., Wickings, E. J. and Schneider, H. P. G. (1979). Suppression of prolactin secretion by lisuride throughout the menstrual cycle and in hyperprolactinaemic menstrual disorders. *Acta Endocrinol.* (Copenhagen), **92**, 78

23. Uilenbroek, J. Th. J., van der Schoot, P., Den Besten, D. and Lankhorst, R. R. (1982). A possible direct effect of prolactin on follicular activity. *Biol. Reprod.*, **27**, 1119

24. Dorrington, J. H. and Gore-Langton, R. E. (1982). Antigonadal action of prolactin: further studies on the mechanism of inhibition of follicle-stimulating hormone-induced aromatase activity in rat granulosa cell cultures. *Endocrinology*, **110**, 1701

25. Erickson, G. F. (1983). Primary cultures of ovarian cells in serum-free medium as models of hormone-dependent differentiation. *Mol. Cell. Endocrinol.*, **29**, 21

26. McNatty, K. P. (1979b). Relationship between plasma prolactin and the endocrine microenvironment of the developing human antral follicle. *Fertil. Steril.*, **32**, 433

27. Nolin, J. M. (1982). Molecular homology between prolactin and ovarian peptides: evidence for physiologic modification of the parent molecule by the target. *Peptides*, **3**, 823

28. Dunaif, A. F., Zimmerman, E. A., Friesen, H. G. and Frantz, A. G. (1982). Intracellular localization of prolactin receptor in the rat ovary by immunocytochemistry. *Endocrinology*, **110**, 1465

29. Dave, J. R., Brown, N. V. and Knázek, R. A. (1982). Prolactin modifies the prostaglandin synthesis, prolactin binding and fluidity of mouse liver membranes. *Biochem. Biophys. Res. Commun.*, **108**, 193

30. McNeilly, A. S. (1980). Prolactin and the control of gonadotrophin secretion in the female. *J. Reprod. Fertil.*, **58**, 537

31

31. Rothschild, I. (1960). The corpus luteum–pituitary relationship: the association between the cause of luteotrophin secretion and the cause of follicular quiescence during lactation. *Endocrinology*, **67**, 9

32. Richardson, D. W., Goldsmith, L. T., Pohl, C. R., Germak, J. A. and Knobil, E. (1982). Is prolactin a luteotrophic hormone in primates? Program of the Endocrine Society Annual Meeting, p. 130 (Suppl. to *Endocrinology*, **110**, 1982)

33. Navickis, R. J., Jones, P. B. C. and Hsueh, A. J. W. (1982). Modulation of prolactin receptors in cultured rat granulosa cells by FSH, LH, and GnRH. *Mol. Cell. Endocrinol.*, **27**, 77

34. Weiss, T. J., Nancarrow, C. D., Armstrong, D. T. and Donnelly, J. B. (1981). Modulation of functional capacity of small ovarian follicles in the post-partum cow by prolactin. *Aust. J. Biol. Sci.*, **34**, 479

35. McNatty, K. P., Sawers, R. S. and McNeilly, A. S. (1974). A possible role for prolactin in control of steroid secretion by the human Graafian follicle. *Nature*, **250**, 653

36. Stouffer, R. L., Coensgen, J. L. and Hodgen, G. D. (1980). Progesterone production by luteal cells isolated from Cynomolgus monkeys: effects of gonadotropin and prolactin during acute incubation and cell culture. *Steroids*, **35**, 523

37. Blackwell, R. E., Boots, L. R. and Potter, H. D. Jr. (1982). Evaluation of delestrogen and parlodel as a luteolytic agent in human. *Fertil. Steril.*, **37**, 213

38. Castracane, V. D. and Goldzieher, J. W. (1982). The luteolytic and abortifacient potential of an estrogen bromergocryptine regimen in the baboon. *Fertil. Steril.*, **37**, 258

39. Lenton, E. A., Sulaiman, R., Sobowale, O. and Cooke, I. D. (1982). The human menstrual cycle: plasma concentrations of prolactin, LH, oestradiol and progesterone in conceiving and non-conceiving women. *J. Reprod. Fertil.*, **65**, 131

40. Andersen, A. N., Hertz, J., Kjer, J. J., Eskildsen, P. C., Larsen, P. S., Svenstrup, B., Nielsen, J. and Arends, J. (1980). Ovarian and placental hormones during prolactin suppression and stimulation in early human pregnancy. *Clin. Endocrinol.*, **13**, 151

41. Ranta, T., Lehtovirta, P., Stenman, U. H., Laatikainen, T. and Seppälä, M. (1980). Acute changes in serum prolactin concentration have no effect on the secretion of progesterone estradiol, or chorionic gonadotropin during early pregnancy. *J. Clin. Endocrinol. Metab.*, **51**, 544

42. Ylikorkala, O., Kivinen, S., Ronnberg, L. and Vinikka, L. (1980). Sulpiride treatment during early human pregnancy: effect on the levels of prolactin, sex steroids, and placental lactogen. *J. Clin. Endocrinol. Metab.*, **51**, 155

43. Tan, G. J. S. and Biggs, J. S. G. (1983). Effects of prolactin on steroid production by human luteal cells in vitro. *J. Endocrinol.*, **96**, 499

44. Vollman, R. (1977). *The Menstrual Cycle*. (Philadelphia: Saunders)

45. Foster, D. L. (1977). Luteinizing hormone and progesterone secretion during sexual maturation of the rhesus monkey: short luteal phases during the initial menstrual cycles. *Biol. Reprod.*, **17**, 584

46. Daily, R. A. and Neill, J. D. (1981). Seasonal variation in reproductive hormones of rhesus monkeys: anovulatory and short luteal phase menstrual cycles. *Biol. Reprod.*, **25**, 250

47. Karsch, F. J., Goodman, R. L. and Legan, S. J. (1980). Feedback basis of seasonal breeding: test of an hypothesis. *J. Reprod. Fertil.*, **58**, 521

48. Haresign, W. and Lamming, G. E. (1978). Comparison of LH release and luteal function in cyclic and LH-RH-treated anoestrous ewes pretreated with PMSG or oestrogen. *J. Reprod. Fertil.*, **52**, 349

49. Land, R. B., Carr, W. R., McNeilly, A. S. and Preece, R. D. (1980). Plasma FSH, LH, the positive feedback of oestrogen, ovulation and luteal function in the ewe given bromocriptine to suppress prolactin during seasonal anoestrus. *J. Reprod. Fertil.*, **59**, 73

50. Pierantoni, R., Genazzani, A. R., Perotti, L., et al. (1983). Plasma levels of luteinizing hormone, estradiol and androstenedione in sows with inadequate plasma progesterone. *J. Endocrinol. Invest.*, **6**, 29

51. Camp, J. C., Wildt, D. E., Howard, P. K., Stuart, L. D. and Chakraborty, P. K. (1983). Ovarian activity during normal and abnormal length estrous cycles in the goat. *Biol. Reprod.*, **28**, 673

52. Rhodes, R. C., III and Randle, R. D. (1979). The effect of season and 5 milligram melatonin administered twice daily on days 14 through 19 of the reproductive cycle of Brahman cows. Program of the 71st Annual Meeting of the American Society of Animal Science, p. 331

53. Poindexter, A. N., III, Ritter, M. B. and Besch, P. K. (1983). The recovery of normal plasma progesterone levels in the post-partum female. *Fertil. Steril.*, **39**, 494
54. Delvoye, P., Delongne-Desnoeck, J. and Robyn, C. (1980). Hyperprolactinaemia during prolonged lactation: evidence for anovulatory cycles and inadequate corpus luteum. *Clin. Endocrinol.*, **13**, 243
55. Caudle, A. B., Thompson, F. N., Purswell, B., Sharlin, J. S., Brooks, P. M. and Smith, C. K. (1982). Effect of monitoring corpus luteum function on days open. *J. Dairy Sci.*, **65**, 638
56. Kindahl, H., Edqvist, L.-E., Larsson, K. and Nalmqvist, A. (1982). Influence of prostaglandins on ovarian function postpartum. In Karg, H. and Schallenberger, E. (eds.) *Factors Influencing Fertility in the Post-Partum Cow*. p. 173. (The Hague: Martinus Nijhoff)
57. Rolland, R., Lequin, R. M., Schellekens, L. A. and De Jong, F. H. (1975). The role of prolactin in the restoration of ovarian function during the early postpartum period in the human female. *Clin. Endocrinol.*, **4**, 15
58. Ducharme, J. F. (1981). Normal puberty: clinical manifestations and their endocrine control. In Collu, R., Ducharme, J. P. and Guyda, H. (eds.) *Pediatric Endocrinology*. p. 293. (New York: Raven Press)
59. Richards, J. S. (1979). Hormonal control of ovarian follicular development: a 1978 perspective. *Recent Prog. Horm. Res.*, **35**, 343
60. Leung, P. C. K. and Armstrong, D. T. (1980). Interactions of steroids and gonadotropins in the control of steroidogenesis in the ovarian follicle. *Ann. Rev. Physiol*, **42**, 71
61. Hillier, S. G. and DeZwart, F. A. (1981). Evidence that granulosa cell aromatase induction/activation by follicle-stimulating hormone is an androgen receptor-regulated process *in-vitro*. *Endocrinology*, **109**, 1303
62. Peluso, J. J., Brown, I. and Steger, R. W. (1979). Effects of cyproterone acetate, a potent anti-androgen, on the preovulatory follicle. *Biol. Reprod.*, **21**, 929
63. Pohl, C. R., Richardson, D. W., Hutchison, J. S. and Knobil, E. (1983). Hypophysiotropic signal for frequency and the functioning of the pituitary–ovarian system in the rhesus monkey. *Endocrinology*, **112**, 2076
64. Terranova, P. F., Martin, N. C. and Chen, S. (1982). Theca is the source of progesterone in experimentally induced atretic follicles of the hamster. *Biol. Reprod.*, **26**, 721
65. Koninckx, P. R. and Brosens, I. A. (1982). The luteinized unruptured follicle syndrome. *Obstet. Gynecol. Ann.*, **11**, 175
66. Auletta, F. J., Kamps, D., Pories, S. and Gibson, M. (1981). Intra-corpus luteum site for the luteolytic action of $PGF_{2\alpha}$ in the rhesus monkey. *Acta Endocrinol.*, **243** (Suppl.), 97
67. Toppozada, M., El-Sokkary, H., El-Abd, M., El-Fazary, A. and El-Rahman, H. A. (1981). Induction of human luteolysis by high dose infusions of 15-methyl $PGF_{2\alpha}$. *Prostaglandins and Med.*, **6**, 203
68. Dennefors, B. L., Sjorgren, A. and Hamberger, L. (1982). Progesterone and adenosine 3′,5′-monophosphate formation by isolated human corpora lutea of different ages: influence of human chorionic gonadotropin and prostaglandins. *J. Clin. Endocrinol. Metab.*, **55**, 102
69. Vijayakumar, R. and Walters, W. A. W. (1983). Human luteal tissue prostaglandins, 17β-estradiol, and progesterone in relation to the growth and senescence of the corpus luteum. *Fertil. Steril.*, **39**, 298
70. Schoonmaker, J. N., Bergman, K. S., Steiner, R. A. and Karsch, F. J. (1982). Estradiol-induced luteal regression in the rhesus monkey: evidence for an extraovarian site of action. *Endocrinology*, **110**, 1708
71. Westfahl, P. K. and King, O. R. (1982). Relationship of estradiol to luteal function in the cycling baboon. *Endocrinology*, **110**, 64
72. Schoonmaker, J. N., Victery, W. and Karsch, F. J. (1981). A receptive period for estradiol-induced luteolysis in the rhesus monkey. *Endocrinology*, **108**, 1874
73. Henderson, K. M. and Franchimont, P. (1981). Regulation of inhibin production by bovine ovarian cells *in vitro*. *J. Reprod. Fertil.*, **63**, 431
74. Rothchild, I. (1965). Interrelationship between progesterone and the ovary, pituitary, and the central nervous system in the control of ovulation, etc. *Vit. Horm.*, **23**, 209
75. Lin, T. J., Billiar, R. B. and Little, B. (1972). Clearance rate of progesterone in the menstrual cycle. *J. Clin. Endocrinol. Metab.*, **35**, 879
76. Nadji, P., Reyniak, J. V., Sedlis, A., Szarowski, D. H. and Bartosik, D. (1975). Endometrial dating correlated with progesterone levels. *Obstet. Gynecol.*, **45**, 193

Discussion

Bettendorf	Is the inadequate corpus luteum an aetiologic entity or is it not just a form of ovarian insufficiency like the other types, e.g. anovulatory cycles or amenorrhea, and do we not have to look for specific causes of inadequate luteal phase?
Rothchild	I do not think that the inadequate corpus luteum is a specific entity in a sense you spoke of, except possibly in association with certain types of anovulation. The most frequent outcome of the interaction between follicles and gonadotropins is no ovulation at all in this particular kind of disturbance. But we also notice this association with a fairly sizeable proportion of cycles where ovulation does occur but is frequently accompanied by a short luteal phase. The other alternative is the possibility that there may be specific causes of formation of an insufficient corpus luteum. I can hardly believe what Dr Taubert pointed out, that 45% of patients with infertility would truly have an inadequate corpus luteum in a sense that this is the reason why they are infertile. And I do not believe that 30% of healthy young volunteer women would have a short luteal phase as it was deduced from the progesterone patterns by Ross in 1970. A perfectly normal woman is entitled to have an anovulatory cycle once a year or once in 2 years. This is a perfectly normal phenomenon, and an inadequate corpus luteum is simply one aspect of this tendency. But otherwise I do not see that we are looking for specific causes for e.g. the Stein–Leventhal syndrome or exercise- or dietary-related anovulation.
Bettendorf	It is an answer, but I think it does not solve the problem, because I speak as a clinician. During puberty and the premenopause you have a continuous transition from the anovulatory stage through maybe the luteal phase defect-stage to normal ovarian function. This can happen to a woman at any time throughout her whole life. The greatest part of our infertility patients have what we call luteal insufficiency, as Dr Taubert mentioned. But I would like to call it insufficient cycle, because we really do not know in any case whether it is a luteal insufficiency.
Rothchild	I really agree completely. The relationship with endometrial defects is probably more important. I think that there are certainly some women whose endometrium does not respond to progesterone. This is a genetic problem and we cannot recognize it from the pattern of progesterone secretion, but only from the endometrium biopsy and/or from the ability of the woman to get pregnant.
Insler	There are rather few women who show corpus luteum insufficiency in each cycle. Most of them have some kind of a cycle disturbance, but which kind manifests itself may be rather a matter of chance. They may have in one cycle corpus luteum insufficiency, the next cycle may be prolonged with a delay of ovulation, and the third one may be anovulatory. I think we are in deep trouble with respect to diagnosis; in the clinic most of the work is actually based on a single parameter which is very bad, and that is the length of the hyperthermic phase.

| | I agree with your remark that hyperprolactinaemia is probably irrele- |

I agree with your remark that hyperprolactinaemia is probably irrelevant. In the past we have observed that in patients treated with hMG/hCG, hyperprolactinaemia did not interfere with the corpus luteum function. Similarly, when we tried to stimulate the insufficient corpus luteum with GnRH in our present study, we observed hyperprolactinaemia in two cases which, however, did not seem to interfere with luteal function.

Rothchild   One of the most important points of my paper is the association between hyperprolactinaemia and the insufficient corpus luteum. This is, however, not due to prolactin but to the association between hyperprolactinaemia and insufficient gonadotropin secretion. That is the reason why treatment of hyperprolactinaemic women improves their gonadotropin secretion. Prolactin probably has an inhibiting effect on gonadotropin secretion through the hypothalamus, but has no effect on the follicle or the corpus luteum.

Wentz   I would like to ask each speaker for his definition of corpus luteum inadequacy.

Schneider   The definition depends on the duration of the luteal phase between ovulation and menstruation, and on the progesterone level on the 7th or 8th day of the luteal phase, whereby ovulation is recognized by ultrasonography and, in some cases, by measuring LH peaks. In a group of 74 patients we identified 41 with corpus luteum insufficiency according to my definition, 28 were hyperprolactinaemic, 4 were hypothyroid, 1 was hyperthyroid, 2 had a PCO syndrome, and 3 had a hypothalamic-ovarian insufficiency. The examination with ultrasonography revealed that regular follicular growth with rupture of the follicle occurred only in 14.8%, irregular follicular growth in another 14.8%, regular follicular growth without rupture in 18.9%, and polycystic degeneration in 10.8%. Therefore, anovulation is an ordinary event in patients who are usually referred to as suffering from corpus luteum insufficiency.

Rothchild   The only way in which one can identify a truly inadequate corpus luteum, will be by having a series of blood samples for progesterone measurements not just in one cycle, but in a series of cycles. I do not think that one can rely on a single or even two samples presumably taken at the peak for a true diagnosis of an inadequate corpus luteum. Nevertheless, I wonder about one of the theoretical causes I had been speculating about, that the inadequate corpus luteum itself causes the following one to be inadequate, too. Progesterone actually enhances the capacity of the pituitary to secrete LH and FSH. If, by chance, the corpus luteum turns out to be inadequate and, therefore, secretes less progesterone, perhaps in the following cycle gonadotropin secretion might be insufficient, and therefore, another inadequate corpus luteum would be formed. I think that in normal women it tends to correct itself through some other compensatory mechanism, but if there are some other kinds of pathology, a woman tends to follow this pattern continuously.

Taubert   We were to define what we call corpus luteum insufficiency. When there is an LH-peak, and I find by laparoscopy a fresh corpus luteum with increased estradiol and progesterone levels in the peritoneal fluid as compared to serum, and when subsequent serum progesterone levels are low, and the endometrial biopsy is inadequate, then I am relatively sure. But what I described is certainly not the routine procedure in Frankfurt.

When comparing basal temperature records with endometrial biopsies, we found in apparently normal hyperthermic phases in about 50% an inadequate corpus luteum. When we talk about normal or abnormal LH levels, we usually refer to single measurements on one day. The problem is, whether we do not miss abnormal patterns by this punctual approach which could be instrumental in causing an inadequate corpus luteum, and which could possibly be recognized by the measurement of the 24-hour pulsatile pattern of LH.

Rothchild	As a clinician and scientist you are constantly faced with the frustration of having to make a diagnosis on the basis of insufficient evidence. There is plenty of evidence that the pulsatile pattern of the gonadotropins, of GnRH and perhaps even of the steroids is very important. The question is, how to apply this clinically, because it is very expensive and time-consuming.
Wentz	Just to make it more difficult: there are now data both in the human and in the monkey to show that progesterone output is not only pulsatile, but it follows very nicely the pulsatile LH activity in the luteal phase.
Gerhard	Thirty per cent of the infertile women who were diagnosed by us as having an inadequate luteal phase, were found to have either a latent hyper-thyroidism, latent hyperprolactinaemia, or increased testosterone or DHEA-S levels. This can be treated successfully by dexamethasone, thyroid hormones, or bromocriptine. I think it is easier to define a normal luteal phase than an abnormal one. There should be at least three pro-gesterone levels above 10 ng/ml, taken at 2-day intervals during the hyper-thermic phase, and an endometrial biopsy which is in-phase. In some cases we have found elevated prolactin levels in the luteal phase with normal estradiol and progesterone, although during the early follicular phase basal prolactin levels were normal. In these patients the pregnancy rate is increased by treatment with bromocriptine.
Rothchild	There is another aspect which has to be mentioned. When measuring normal or elevated hormone patterns by RIA, we tend to forget that there is not necessarily a correlation with bioactivity. The gonadotropins and other pituitary hormones are no single chemically defined entities as in the case of steroids, but families of hormones ranging in bioactivity over a whole spectrum of effects. Some of the cases of infertility may go back eventually to pituitary hormones which look normal but do not have the full biological qualities. So they may influence the response of the corpus luteum to hormones secreted by the implanting blastocyst, the secretion of estradiol and progesterone, and the response of the endometrium to progesterone.
Braendle	When we treated FSH deficiency as a cause of insufficient cycle with pure FSH during the first days of follicular phase, we were not able to induce a normal ovulatory cycle, but we succeeded when using hMG. Patients with insufficient cycles showed a higher LH/FSH ratio as compared to normal women. When measuring the pulsatile pattern of LH, we found in insuf-ficient cycles high frequent LH pulses during the early follicular phase which continued during the late follicular phase. In normal cycles the frequency of LH pulses does not increase before the late follicular phase. This could possibly be the result of a progesterone deficiency in the pre-ceding cycle. When we supplemented insufficient cycles with progesterone, we found a decrease of the frequency of LH pulses during the medication.
Rothchild	There is some experimental evidence that progesterone treatment of the anestrus sheep along with gonadotropin or GnRH results in a corpus luteum that behaves like a normal one. Looking at the literature I am impressed by the high incidence of cures of presumably inadequate corpus luteum as a cause of infertility with progesterone treatment. Possibly the progesterone treatment itself corrects the tendency of the following cycle to be insufficient.
L'Hermite	I would like to add some remarks with respect to prolactin. Hyperpro-lactinaemia probably does not act at the ovarian level or at least does not have any direct major inhibitory influence. However, it affects gonado-tropin secretion. I must criticize what was said in the paper of McNatty *et al.* cited by Dr. Rothchild. They stated that steroidogenesis was im-paired, while what they showed was a reduced progesterone secretion by granulosa cells which were luteinized *in vitro*. The other paper of McNatty *et al.* I want to criticize is where they collected follicles by laparotomy and

tried to correlate the prolactin levels at the time of operation to the granulosa cell activity. They did not have enough data on the endocrine environment during the preceding weeks, or at least days, before operation, and there was a stressful situation with drugs being given for premedication and possibly for anaesthesia which could influence the prolactin levels. But I would like to question Dr Gerhard about the increased prolactin in the luteal phase despite normal progesterone. I wonder whether this could not be just the result of an increased estradiol production when you overstimulate for ovulation induction. But this does not interfere at all with the development of corpus luteum function or pregnancy. When you claim that bromocriptine treatment increases pregnancy rate, I would like to ask whether these data are really formally established by double-blind study or something like that. Our investigations a few years ago on bromocriptine treatment of normoprolactinaemic patients in controlled studies revealed no improvement. I also wonder whether the prolactin produced by the endometrium would reach the general circulation and so would account for the increase in the prolactin levels.

Gerhard   If you give bromocriptine to women with normal prolactin levels during the luteal phase, the luteal phase tends to get worse. But if they are hyperprolactinaemic with prolactin levels above 15 ng/ml during the luteal phase, you can increase the pregnancy rate when bromocriptine is given in a dose just sufficient to decrease the prolactin to levels between 5 and 15 ng/ml. When you use clomiphene or gonadotropins for the treatment of luteal phase insufficiency or anovulation, you have an increase in prolactin in about 30% of the patients. In these cases you can increase the pregnancy rate by additional treatment with bromocriptine, too.

Insler   We did not observe significant changes in prolactin levels under clomiphene or gonadotropins. When we tried to treat the spiking in mild luteal phase hyperprolactinaemia with bromocriptine, we could not prove any increase in pregnancy rate. Infertile women, particularly those who are continuously menstruating, may eventually conceive whether or not we treat them, and whatever type of treatment they receive. You must have a controlled cross-over study to prove an increase of the pregnancy rate.

Bettendorf   Dr Gerhard, you always say you have a higher pregnancy rate; what is the absolute figure?

Gerhard   I cannot tell you at this moment because we conduct this as a prospective study.

Bettendorf   Then you cannot say you have a higher rate unless you can present figures.

3
Induced luteal defect after follicle aspiration?

F. LEHMANN, K. DIEDRICH, H. VAN DER VEN, S. AL-HASANI,
CH. SCHULZ AND D. KREBS

In earlier studies we could show that after stimulation with clomiphene, 100 mg per day from day 5 to 9, the luteal progesterone plasma concentrations were not lowered by follicular aspiration[1] (Figure 3.1). These findings were in concordance with the results of other groups, who also worked on an *in vitro* fertilization (IVF) programme[2-4].

Since these studies were performed we have changed the scheme of ovarian stimulation, in that we administered 150 mg instead of 100 mg Clomid per

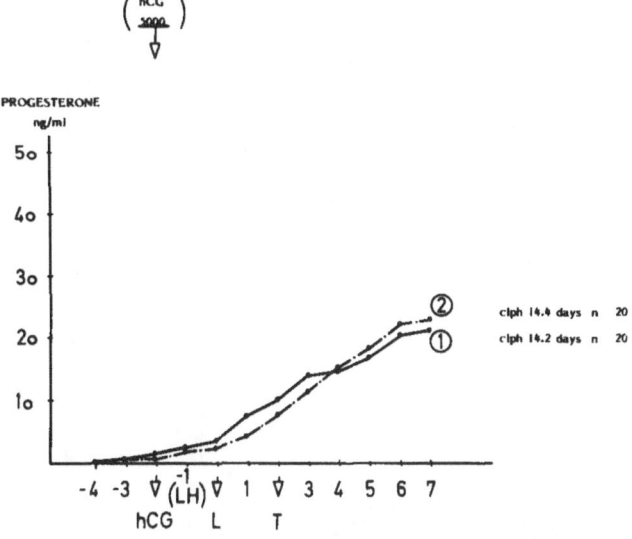

Figure 3.1 Plasma progesterone concentrations. 1: Clomiphene 2 × 50 mg day 5–9, no hCG, no laparoscopy; 2: clomiphene 2 × 50 mg day 5–9, 5000 IU hCG, follicular aspiration. L = Laparoscopy; T = transfer

39

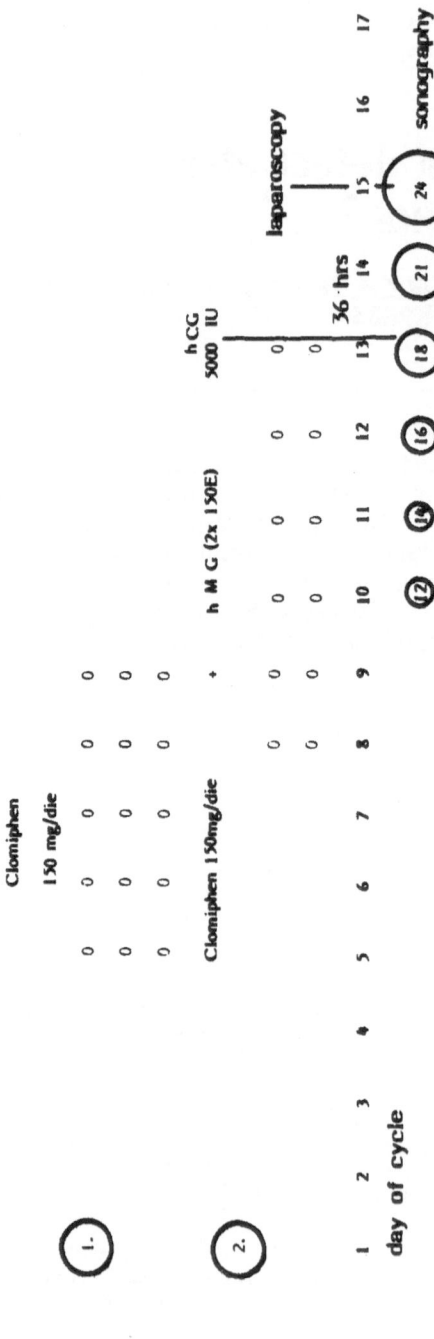

Figure 3.2 Therapeutic regimes for *in vitro* fertilization (IVF) and embryo transfer (ET). **1:** Clomiphene 3 × 50 mg day 5–9; **2:** clomiphene 3 × 50 mg day 5–9, continued by 4 ampoules hMG per day until hCG administration

day from day 5 to day 9 of the cycle, and then combined the clomiphene therapy with injections of hMG (Figure 3.2). The more intensive stimulation was expected to lead to an increase in the recovery of oocytes, and to a transfer (ET) of a larger number of embryos per trial. Although this aim seemed to be within reach, the pregnancy rate did not increase as expected; in addition many of the induced pregnancies ended in an abortion.

We therefore felt that we had to re-evaluate the corpus luteum phase after introducing this new and very intensive approach to ovarian stimulation as a possible limiting factor in the induction of pregnancies in our IVF and ET programme.

When we measured the estradiol (E_2) and the progesterone (P) levels in spontaneous cycles and also after clomiphene therapy (100 and 150 mg per day) we found that the estradiol levels in the luteal phase of the two therapy groups reached the same percentage of the periovulatory peak values as in spontaneous cycles, whereas the progesterone concentration did not reach the expected levels as had been calculated from the E_2 peak values (Figures 3.3 and 3.4).

This relative progesterone deficiency could be readjusted to a progesterone/estradiol ratio comparable to that of spontaneous cycles by administration of additional hCG on day 3 and 8 after the laparoscopy (Figures 3.5 and 3.6).

The combined clomiphene/hMG treatment brought about an enormous change of the course of E_2 and P concentrations in plasma which differed considerably from that of spontaneous cycles. The relative progesterone

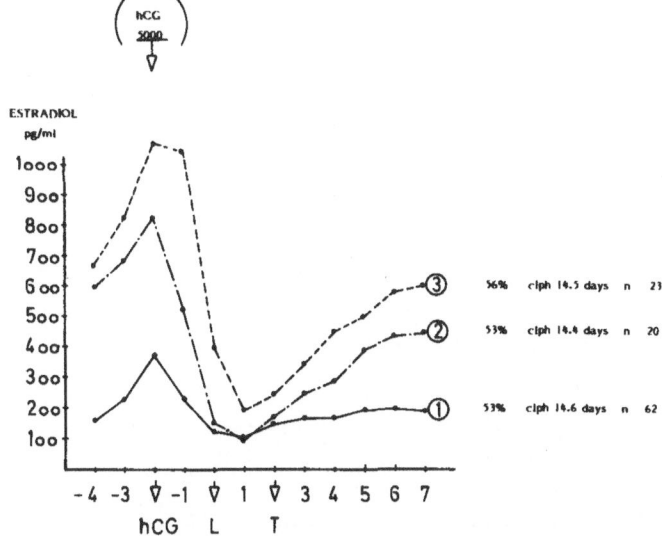

Figure 3.3 Plasma estradiol concentrations. 1: In spontaneous cycles; 2: after clomiphene 2 × 50 mg day 5–9 and 5000 IU hCG; 3: after clomiphene 3 × 50 mg day 5–9 and 5000 IU hCG. Mean values and percentages of mid-luteal concentrations in relation to periovulatory estradiol peak. clph = Corpus luteum phase

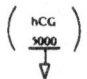

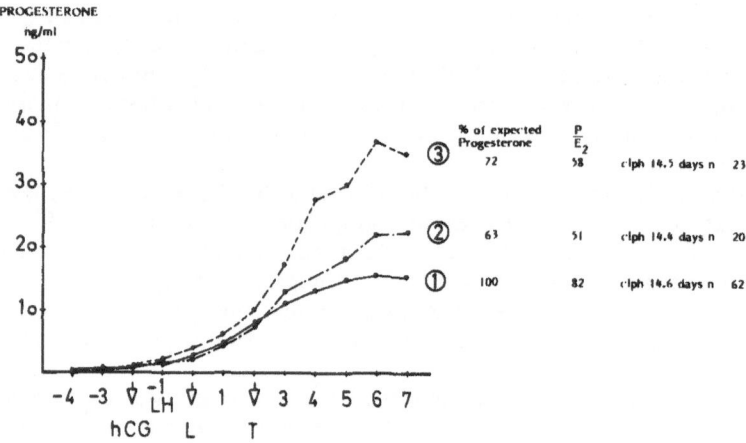

Figure 3.4 Plasma progesterone concentrations. 1: In spontaneous cycles; 2: after clomiphene 2×50 mg day 5–9 and 5000 IU hCG; 3: after clomiphene 3×50 mg day 5–9 and 5000 IU hCG. Mean values and percentages in relation to periovulatory estradiol peak. clph = Corpus luteum phase

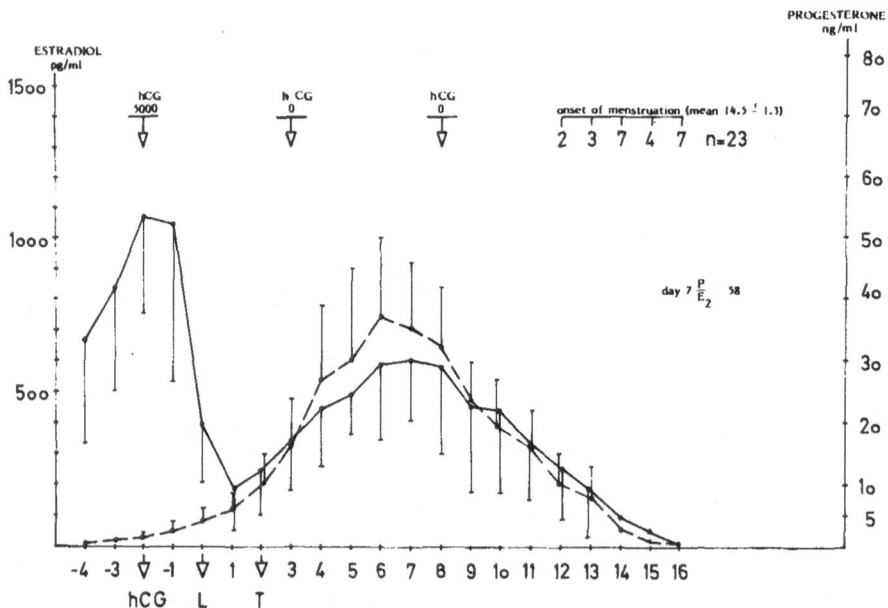

Figure 3.5 Ovarian stimulation with clomiphene 3×50 mg day 5–9, no hCG administration in the luteal phase

42

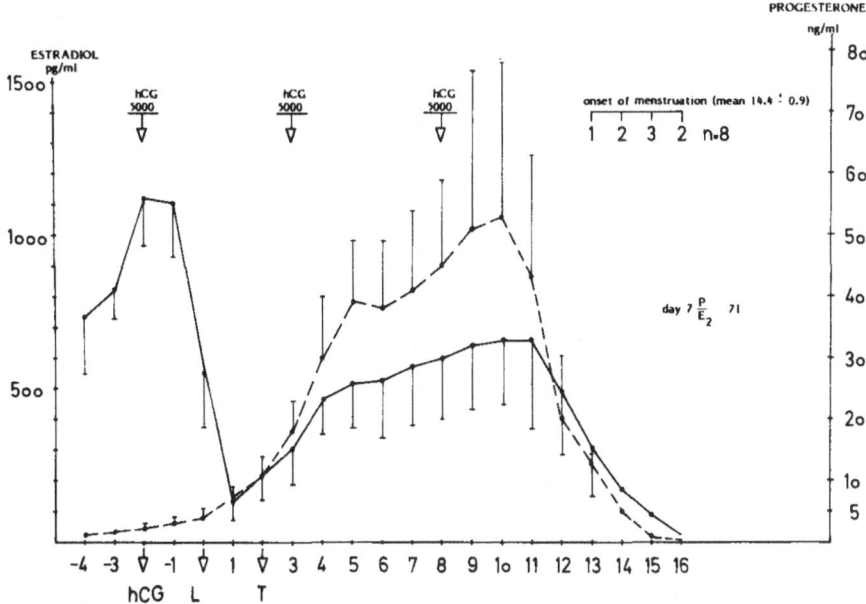

Figure 3.6 Ovarian stimulation with clomiphene 3×50 mg day 5–9, hCG administration on day 3 and 8 of the luteal phase

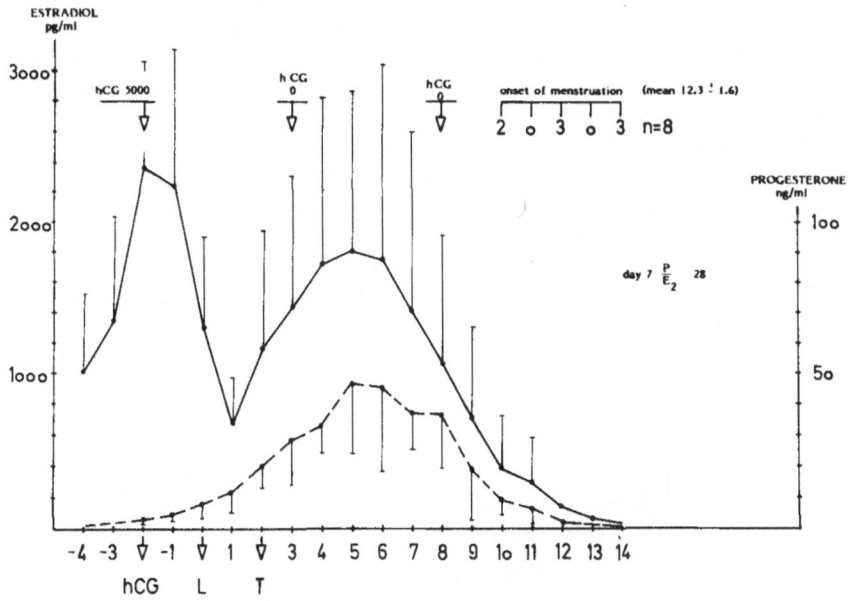

Figure 3.7 Ovarian stimulation with clomiphene 3×50 mg day 5–9 continued by gonadotropins, no hCG administration in the luteal phase

43

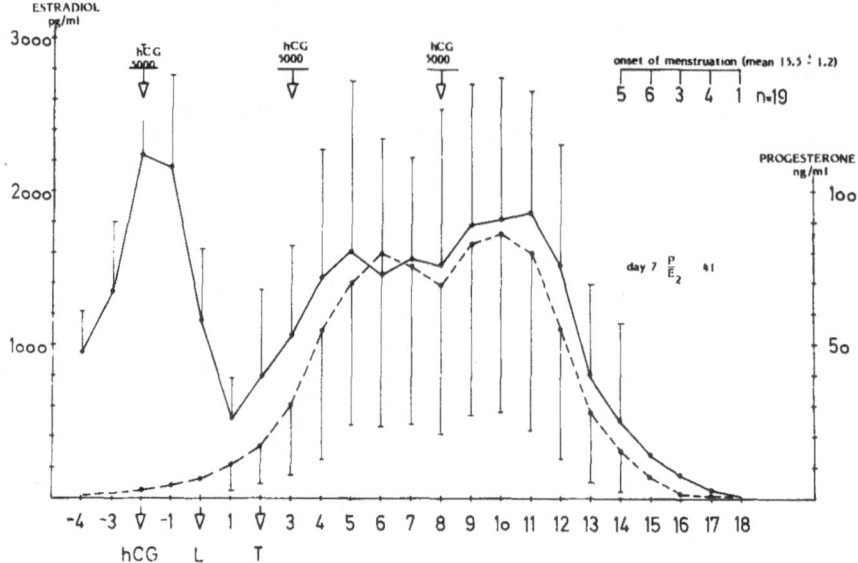

Figure 3.8 Ovarian stimulation with clomiphene 3×50 mg day 5–9 continued by gonado-tropins, hCG administration on day 3 and 8 of the luteal phase

deficiency in the middle of the luteal phase (mean P/E_2 ratio 28; Figure 3.7) was found to be much more pronounced as compared to the results of the administration of 150 mg clomiphene (mean P/E_2 ratio 58; Figure 3.5) or to the values in normal cycles (mean P/E_2 ratio 82). hCG administration on day 3 and 8 after laparoscopy resulted in a double increase of P values, whereas the E_2 concentrations increased only a little (Figure 3.8).

The mean values of the P/E_2 ratios and absolute values of P after clomi-phene and clomiphene/hMG stimulation on day 7 of the luteal phase – the assumed day of implantation – are summarized in Tables 3.1 and 3.2 in relation to luteal hCG therapy.

The need for additional hCG therapy in the luteal phase became evident when the clomiphene/hMG therapy was applied, whereas the high-dosage

Table 3.1 Quotient of progesterone (P) and estradiol (E_2) on day 7 of the luteal phase after clomiphene-stimulation (day 5–9). Role of luteal hCG therapy. Mean values

n	Therapy	Day 7 P/E_2	P (ng/ml) plasma values on day 7
23	Clomiphene 3×50 mg no luteal hCG	58	35
8	Clomiphene 3×50 mg 2×5000 hCG	71	41
12	Clomiphene 3×50 mg 10×1000 hCG	85	53
—	Clomiphene 3×50 mg no luteal hCG, pregnancy	71	50
62	Spontaneous cycles	82	15

Table 3.2 Quotient of progesterone (P) and estradiol (E$_2$) on day 7 of the luteal phase after clomiphene/hMG-stimulation (day 5–9 and 8 until hCG). Role of luteal hCG therapy. Mean values

n	Therapy	Day 7 P/E$_2$	P (ng/ml) plasma values on day 7
8	Clomiphene/hMG, no luteal hCG	26	37
19	Clomiphene/hMG 2×5000 hCG	41	75
14	Clomiphene/hMG 10×1000 hCG	42	92
1	Clomiphene/hMG 2×5000 hCG, pregnancy	56	98
62	Spontaneous cycles	82	15

clomiphene therapy very frequently resulted in a sufficient luteal function compatible with implantation (Tables 3.3 and 3.4). Low mid-luteal progesterone plasma levels seemed to be followed by abortive implantation. P/E$_2$ ratios higher than 50 on day 7 of the luteal phase may be the prerequisite for an implantation regardless of the outcome of the pregnancy.

Table 3.3 Pregnancies after clomiphene therapy, IVF and ET. Quotient of progesterone (P) and estradiol (E$_2$) on day 7 of the luteal phase and outcome of pregnancies. Role of luteal hCG therapy

No.	Patient	Luteal hCG therapy	Day 7 P/E$_2$	Absolute values on day 7 P (ng/ml)	Clinical performance
1	Sim	2×5000	95	61	born singleton
2	Sch	2×5000	88	77	intact twins
3	Uml	—	60	47	intact singleton
4	Sen	—	54	81	intact singleton
5	Kan	—	50	19	abortion 12th week
6	Die	—	70	31	abortion 7th week

Table 3.4 Pregnancies after clomiphene/hMG therapy, IVF and ET. Quotient of progesterone (P) and estradiol (E$_2$) on day 7 of the luteal phase and outcome of pregnancies. Role of luteal hCG therapy

No.	Patient	Luteal hCG therapy	Day 7 P/E$_2$	Absolute values on day 7 P (ng/ml)	Clinical performance
1	Hen	2×5000	57	130	born singleton
2	Wuc	2×5000	68	68	intact singleton
3	Nai	2×5000	53	95	intact twins
4	Fre	2×5000	51	102	intact twins
5	Pag	2×5000	58	68	abortion 9th week
6	Hei	2×5000	50	50	abortion 6th week (twins)
7	Hof	—	51	30	abortion 6th week (twins)

CONCLUSIONS

(1) The laparoscopic aspiration of preovulatory follicles for IVF and ET does *not* necessarily lead to luteal insufficiency.

(2) Intensive ovarian stimulation induces the development of several generations of follicles. An inadequate luteal phase is the logical consequence, as there is a direct relationship between the number of small, unripe follicles at the time of follicular aspiration, and the existence of a 'relative' deficiency of progesterone which can be detected in the luteal phase.

(3) The progesterone plasma concentrations in such deficient luteal phase can be increased either by exogenous progesterone as proposed by Jones *et al.*[5] or by hCG therapy. The progesterone administration is difficult to guide in terms of needed and actually reached plasma values. The hCG therapy elevates both the estradiol and progesterone plasma levels, even though this is not always needed.

(4) Both the plasma progesterone concentration determined in the first days of the luteal phase until the day of assumed implantation, and the P/E_2 ratio on that day may be helpful parameters in characterizing the effect of circulating steroids on the endometrium. On the basis of therapy cycles which have been evaluated by both parameters, we feel that the absolute values of progesterone are of more importance.

(5) Lower normal values for the P/E_2 ratio which are still compatible with implantation could be defined.

(6) When the ovarian stimulation results in the development of several follicles of the same size, there is little evidence that a luteal phase defect will develop after stimulation with clomiphene.

(7) One possible approach to this problem would be a reduction of the clomiphene dose; another approach would be the use of gonadotropins according to the Norfolk regimen. This type of therapy is characterized by beginning therapy early in the cycle and by a relatively short period of stimulation with exogenous gonadotropins followed by a 60 h period without any further hMG treatment until hCG is administered.

(8) The low-dose clomiphene therapy does not require any additional stimulation of the corpus luteum, if previous spontaneous cycles were normal.

Stimulation with gonadotropins (Norfolk scheme) has to be complemented by the application of progesterone or hCG in the luteal phase, even if all aspirated follicles had reached the preovulatory stage, because endogenous LH production is not sufficient for the high number of receptor sites[6].

hCG therapy could be of advantage as compared to progesterone in these situations, as both estradiol and progesterone will be increased in a physiological relationship.

References

1. Lehmann, F., Diedrich, K., van der Ven, H., Al-Hasani, S. and Krebs, D. (1983). Die Lutealphase nach Follikelpunktion. *Geburtshilfe Frauenheilkd.*, **43**, 305
2. Feichtinger, W., Kemeter, P., Szalay, S., Beck, A. and Janisch, H. (1982). Could aspiration of the Graafian follicle cause luteal phase deficiency? *Fertil. Steril.*, **37**, 205
3. Lopata, A. (1980). Success and failures in human *in vitro* fertilization. *Nature*, **288**, 642
4. Trotnow, S., Becker, H., Kniewald, T., Al-Hasani, S. and Mulz, D. (1982). Luteal phase following oocyte aspiration, *in-vitro* fertilization and embryo transfer in clomid/hCG stimulated cycles. *Arch. Gynaecol.*, **231**, 175
5. Jones, H. W., Jones, G. S., Andrews, M. C., Bundren, C., Garcia, J., Sandow, B., Veeck, L., Wilkens, Ch., Witmyer, J., Wortham, J. E. and Wright, G. (1982). The program for *in vitro* fertilization at Norfolk. *Fertil. Steril.*, **38**, 14
6. Jones, H. W. (1983). Factors influencing implantation and maintenance of pregnancy following embryo transfer. In Beier, H. M. and Lindner, H. R. (eds.) *Fertilization of the Human Egg in Vitro*. pp. 293–301. (Berlin: Springer)

Discussion

Insler   You have women for *in vitro* fertilization who are continuously ovulating. After treatment with ovulation-inducing agents and all these multiple ovulations, this may not be the best group, because you are interfering with the cycle. The group with hypogonadotropic amenorrhoea may be better for ovulation-induction because you are starting with nothing. My question is: you did not observe a reduction of progesterone levels after follicle aspiration. This is in contrast to the report of Jones, who counted the number of flushings. What was the number of flushings in your series?

Lehmann   It is our concept to perform an embryo transfer with at least two or three embryos, and therefore we change the physiological condition into an unphysiological one. Follicle aspiration imposes the question of how to manage the problem of a luteal phase which is not comparable to a luteal phase insufficiency of a spontaneous cycle. We do not really flush, but rather empty the follicle very gently in order to withdraw as few as possible granulosa cells with the fluid. There is no flushing even if we miss the egg.

Rothchild   Jones counted the number of flushes, but there was no correlation between the number of granulosa cells they removed and a formation of an inadequate corpus luteum, although they found lower progesterone levels. The patients with inadequate corpus luteum could have had very few granulosa cells removed, while patients with normal corpus luteum could have had removed a lot of granulosa cells.

Wentz   Unfortunately, we have to go into tremendous detail when you try to interpret granulosa cell experiments. Jones did not differentiate between those follicles which were preovulatory and those that were not; and so she had a mixture of cells under these circumstances.

Lehmann   If you are talking only about one ripe pre-ovulatory follicle and how you work on this, then you have to face the consequences in the luteal phase. It is quite a different situation as compared to the one you have after gonadotropin stimulation, where you have follicles sized between 10 and 24 mm diameter. If you flush one or two of them because you missed the egg, you probably will not see any difference in the progesterone level in the luteal phase due to the large number of corpora lutea. But if there was only one big follicle and you lose all the granulosa cells of this follicle, progesterone secretion will be appreciably affected.

On the other hand, the more we stimulate, the more we are apt to get a relative progesterone deficiency in the luteal phase, because you have follicles after aspiration which cannot take over progesterone synthesis just like an aspirated pre-ovulatory follicle. So what you are really doing is to mix a population of follicles, and the same applies to the secretory pattern in the succeeding luteal phase. You may achieve a pregnancy with fertilized oocytes from various follicles, but the one which then is transferred, may be supported for the implantation by the corpus luteum of a large follicle where you missed the egg.

4
Role of prolactin in the pathogenesis of the human inadequate luteal phase

M. L'HERMITE

It is well established that, in most laboratory animal species, prolactin (PRL) is the luteotropic hormone. On the contrary, clinical and experimental data are much less convincing in the human, in whom luteinizing hormone (LH) clearly exerts a luteotropic activity. We will therefore review the present status of our knowledge concerning the potential role of prolactin in the pathogenesis of the inadequate luteal phase.

HYPERPROLACTINAEMIA-ASSOCIATED INADEQUATE LUTEAL PHASES

Besides the well-known causal relationship between hyperprolactinaemia and amenorrhoea (with or without galactorrhoea), we[1], as well as others (as reviewed recently[2]), reported the occurrence of short and/or inadequate luteal phases in infertile hyperprolactinaemic patients. Despite the fact that an endocrinologically normal menstrual cycle can occur exceptionally despite sustained hyperprolactinaemia[3], it has even been proposed that the hyper-prolactinaemic short luteal phase cycle might represent an early stage of the hyperprolactinaemic amenorrhoea syndrome[4]. Bromocriptine (or lisuride in some cases) administration normalized PRL levels and usually corrected the short or inadequate luteal phase. However, from the survey[2] of published series, an overall pregnancy rate of 38% (out of 50 cases) is far from being very convincing. Despite the need for a more careful assessment of the efficacy of dopaminergic drugs in the treatment of the infertility of patients with hyperprolactinaemia-associated inadequate luteal phase, most clinicians nowadays accept the causal relationship and the indication of a dopaminergic treatment for infertility in any case of sustained hyperprolactinaemia.

Conflicting reports have, however, been published. Thus Sarris et al.[5] described a group of 39 women with elevated PRL but normal progesterone mid-luteal levels, whose infertility failed to be improved by bromocriptine over more than 9 months; it was, however, impossible from their data to ascertain that these women had sustained hyperprolactinaemia rather than elevation of PRL only during the luteal phase and/or possibly in relation to some kind of stress. In a group of 36 infertile women with short luteal phase (as evaluated planimetrically from the basal body temperature curve chart), Fredricsson et al.[6] found somewhat higher PRL and lower progesterone mid-luteal levels; furthermore, bromocriptine administered in a double-blind fashion failed to affect progesterone levels and 6 out of 7 conceptions obtained did occur during placebo administration. Finally, one should mention the work of Vanrell and Balasch[7], who detected hyperprolactinaemia in 15 out of 130 infertile patients (i.e. 11.5%) with regular menstrual cycles; they reported similar luteal phase lengths and progesterone levels in their hyper-prolactinaemic than in the normoprolactinaemic patients. Furthermore, a significantly higher incidence, of histologically documented inadequate luteal phase, was documented in the normoprolactinaemic group. All these reports do not exclude that hyperprolactinaemia can, when sustained, induce infertility through inadequate luteal function; they point out, however, that there is little – if any – correlation between PRL and progesterone in the luteal phase, and that the usefulness of PRL measurement is scanty in the evaluation of luteal function in infertility.

PROLACTIN AND THE NORMAL LUTEAL PHASE

From the above discussion it appears that high levels of PRL can be luteolytic in the human in pathological conditions, but PRL is unlikely to exert physiologically such a role. The only *in vivo* evidence, that PRL might be required for normal luteal function, comes from the work of Schulz et al.[8]: these authors recorded markedly decreased progesterone levels in the luteal phase of women treated, for the entire length of their menstrual cycle, with doses of bromocriptine sufficient to suppress PRL to below-normal levels. It is, however, not excluded that bromocriptine may, through its dopaminergic activity, have acted upon gonadotropin secretion to modify luteal function, rather than via inhibition of PRL secretion.

These *in vivo* data have to be compared with caution to the scarce *in vitro* data obtained in the human. Initially McNatty et al.[9] concluded that high PRL levels might inhibit follicular steroidogenesis; they observed in fact an impairment of progesterone secretion by luteinized follicular cells submitted to high local concentrations of PRL, but failed to evidence any clear correlation between intrafollicular and circulating PRL concentrations. Later, McNatty[10] demonstrated an association between high levels of intrafollicular PRL and a marked reduction in FSH accumulation, together with low levels of estradiol in antral fluid. Such an elevation of intrafollicular fluid was observed only when plasma PRL levels (unfortunately determined only once, just before ovariectomy!) were exceeding 100 ng/ml; there was also a severe deficiency in granulosa cells of these follicles, but this marked reduction in intrafollicular activity was not associated with any significant changes in peripheral FSH and estradiol levels. Thus there appears to be some relationship between highly elevated PRL blood levels, the endocrine microenvironment and the development of the human antral follicle: hyper-prolactinaemia could impair luteal function by this mechanism rather than by a direct effect upon the corpus luteum.

INTERFERENCE WITH THE HUMAN MENSTRUAL CYCLE BY CHRONIC DRUG-INDUCED HYPERPROLACTINAEMIA

Since it is impossible, in hyperprolactinaemic patients, to follow the hormonal events occurring from the very onset of hyperprolactinaemia, we[11] analysed the hormonal and menstrual patterns of normal volunteer women receiving benzamides (sulpiride, tiapride or metoclopramide) at dosages and schedules adequate to induce a sustained hyperprolactinaemia[12, 13]. Benzamides act directly at the level of the pituitary to counteract the inhibitory effect of dopamine[14]; furthermore, their hypothalamic effects are apparently entirely dependent on the resulting hyperprolactinaemia[15]. Recent animal data[16] indicate that sulpiride induced an increase in pituitary LH and FSH contents, as well as in the LH-RH concentrations and dopamine turnover within the mediobasal hypothalamus. When sulpiride or tiapride was administered continuously from the onset of the menstrual cycle for 2–3 cycles (or their equivalent), a progressive deterioration occurred, from short luteal phase cycles to anovulatory cycles or even amenorrhoea[11, 17].

Figures 4.1 and 4.2 depict the mean levels of LH, FSH, estradiol and progesterone, as well as the mean FSH/LH ratios in, respectively, short luteal phase cycles and anovulatory 'cycles' observed during sulpiride treatment and compared to the control cycles observed in the same subjects. It can be deduced that: (1) there was a lack of impairment of follicular estradiol secretion; (2) gonadotropins (especially LH) were impaired in the luteal phase; (3) the positive feedback of estradiol on LH might have been impaired in the short luteal phase cycles and was clearly abnormal in the anovulatory cycles; (4) modifications of FSH/LH ratios occurred throughout sulpiride administration, although not statistically significant until the luteal phase in short luteal phase cycles.

It has been demonstrated that hyperprolactinaemia is associated with an impaired positive feedback of estrogens and that their negative feedback might even be potentiated[18, 19]. This impaired positive feedback can be overcome with a greater dose of estrogens[20] and is clearly not due to a decreased pituitary gonadotropin reserve[18, 21]. All these data therefore suggest a hypo-thalamic impact of hyperprolactinaemia, disturbing the pulsatile secretion of hypothalamic LH-RH, possibly via an increased dopamine turnover[22], together with an increased opioid activity[23]. The demonstration, by Leyendecker et al.[27], that ovulation can be induced, in hyperprolactinaemic amenorrhoeic patients, by use of pulsatile administration of LH-RH, further supports the hypothesis that hyperprolactinaemia primarily interferes with the pulsatile hypothalamic secretion of LH-RH. It is conceivable that a slight perturbation of the FSH/LH ratio will result, and that this might lead to luteal phase defects[25].

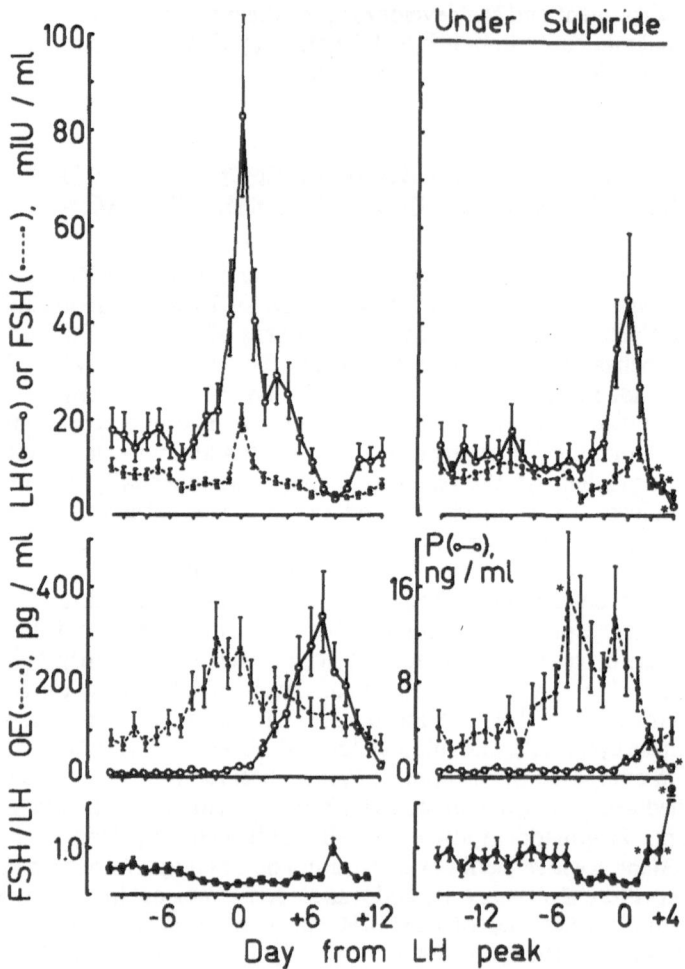

Figure 4.1 Mean (± SE) serum levels of LH, FSH, estradiol (OE) and progesterone (P), as well as mean (± SE) FSH/LH ratios in control cycles (on the left) and in short luteal phase cycles during sulpiride-induced hyperprolactinaemia (on the right). The asterisks indicate mean values that were significantly (at least $p < 0.05$) different in the short luteal phase cycles than the corresponding values in the control cycles. From L'Hermite et al.[17]

In a recent paper, Kauppila et al.[26] followed, by echography, the morphology of the ovarian follicles in seven women in whom hyperprolactinaemia was induced over two consecutive cycles by oral administration of metoclopramide from the 2nd to the 22nd cycle day. They evidenced an abnormal follicular morphological maturation in nine of the 14 treated cycles, consisting of: the appearance of multiple follicles with retarded growth, lack of selection of the dominant follicle, and much-reduced peak diameters of the largest follicles. Because of the latter finding, Kauppila et al. postulated that

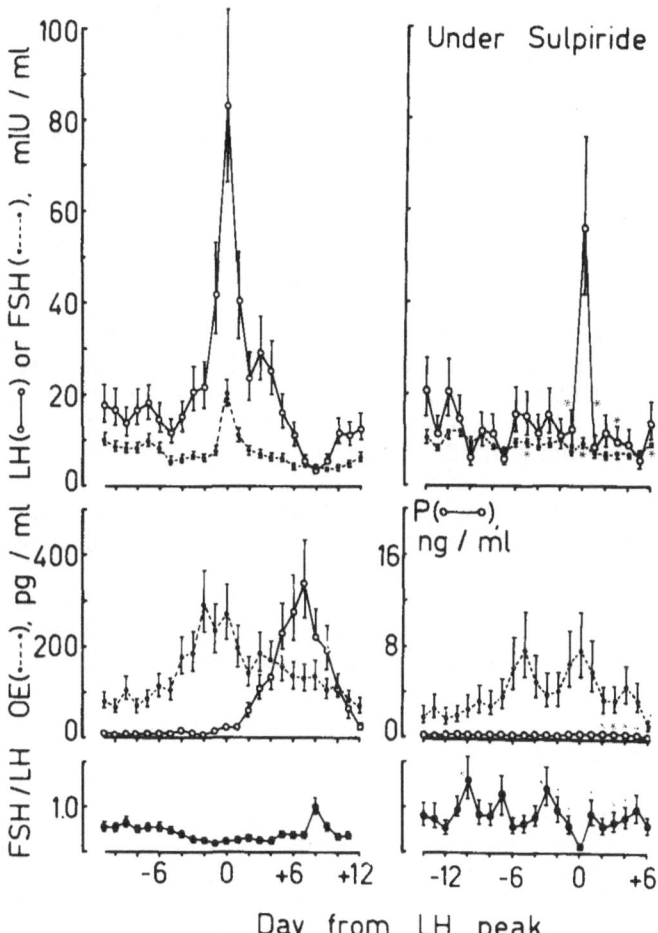

Figure 4.2 Mean (± SE) serum levels of LH, FSH, estradiol (OE) and progesterone (P), as well as mean (± SE) FSH/LH ratios in control cycles (on the left) and in anovulatory cycles under sulpiride-induced hyperprolactinaemia (on the right). The anovulatory cycles were combined according to the day of the major LH burst following or concomitant to some peak estradiol concentration. The asterisks indicate mean values that were significantly (at least $p < 0.05$) different in the anovulatory cycles than the corresponding values in the control cycles. From L'Hermite et al.[17]

these hyperprolactinaemic cycles might in fact have been anovulatory, despite the observation of luteal phases with decreased progesterone secretion. Although this hypothesis had not been investigated by Kauppila et al., Coutts et al.[27], after having monitored ovarian ultrasonography throughout the cycle, reported a definite association between retained luteal phase cysts and the deficient luteal phase. These data, again, are not incompatible with a primary hypothalamic impact of hyperprolactinaemia on LH-RH secretion.

An additional effect, directly at the pituitary level, is possible since Cheung[28] observed, *in vitro* in the animal, an inhibitory effect of PRL on LH release, both in basal as well as stimulated (LH-RH) conditions.

BROMOCRIPTINE TREATMENT IN NORMOPROLACTINAEMIC AMENORRHOEA AND INFERTILITY

In studies using the model of drug-induced hyperprolactinaemia it was shown that hyperprolactinaemia, in order to exert major deleterious effects upon the menstrual cycle, had to be sustained and initiated early in the cycle[11, 17, 21, 26, 29, 30]. A transient hyperprolactinaemia over the mid-cycle period was, however, reported to be associated with shorter luteal phases[31]. Similarly, Ben-David and Schenker[32] identified, among women with regular menstrual cycles but long-standing idiopathic infertility, a subgroup exhibiting transitory PRL elevations for 1–3 days simultaneously to the pre-ovulatory estradiol peak. Since Lenton *et al.*[33] observed lower PRL levels with no increase at mid-cycle in cycles in which conception occurred, in contrast to non-conception cycles, one can conceive that mild and transient hyperprolactinaemia, occurring at the proper time, might somehow interfere with fertility processes.

Although it had been earlier claimed that bromocriptine was successful in the treatment of normoprolactinaemic amenorrhoea, as well as unexplained infertility, double-blind controlled trials failed to confirm it[34–36].

ENDOMETRIAL PROLACTIN AND INADEQUATE LUTEAL FUNCTION

It has been recently demonstrated *in vitro* that human endometrium does synthesize prolactin, and that this synthesis is correlated with the appearance and degree of synthesis and decidualization of the stroma[37, 39]. In addition, Daly *et al.*[39] have observed that samples of luteal phase defect endometrium produced significantly less PRL than did control tissues of the same ideal menstrual dates. It is presently impossible to assess whether this might merely be the consequence of the luteal defect or related to its cause. One could also have proposed that endometrial PRL might contribute to circulating PRL concentrations and, for example, result in elevated PRL levels in the luteal phase. However, data reported by Braendle in the discussion of this workshop (p. 59) suggest that endometrial PRL is not secreted in the general circulation.

Acknowledgments

Part of the work reported here (ref. 17) had been performed in the Human Reproduction Unit of the Department of Obstetrics/Gynaecology of the University Hospital Saint-Pierre. The financial support of the Fonds Emile Defay (Université Libre de Bruxelles) and the secretarial work of Mrs. C. Bekaert are gratefully acknowledged.

References

1. L'Hermite, M., Caufriez, A., Badawi, M., Sugar, J., Schwers, J., Robyn, C., Cordova, T., Ayalon, D., Legros, J. J. and Stévenaert, A. (1978). Selected aspects of hyperprolactinaemia and its management. In Robyn, C. and Harter, M. (eds) *Progress in Prolactin Physiology and Pathology.* pp. 397–414. (Amsterdam: Elsevier/North Holland)
2. Michel, P. St. and diZerega, G. S. (1983). Hyperprolactinaemia and luteal phase dysfunction infertility. *Obstet. Gynecol. Survey*, **38**, 248
3. Tambascia, M., Bahamondes, L., Pinotti, J., Collier, A. M., Dachs, J. N. and Faundes, A. (1980). Sustained hyperprolactinaemia in a normally menstruating woman with apparently normal ovarian function. *Fertil. Steril.*, **34**, 282
4. Bahamondes, L., Saboya, W., Tambascia, M. and Trevisan, M. (1979). Galactorrhea, infertility and short luteal phases in hyperprolactinaemic women: early stage of amenorrhea-galactorrhea? *Fertil. Steril.*, **32**, 476
5. Sarris, S., Swyer, G. I. M., McGarrigle, H. H. G., Lawrence, D. M., Little, V. and Lachelin, G. C. L. (1978). Prolactin and luteal insufficiency. *Clin. Endocrinol.*, **9**, 543
6. Fredricsson, B., Carlström, K., Björk, G. and Messinis, I. (1981). Effects of prolactin and bromocriptine on the luteal phase in infertile women. *Eur. J. Obstet. Gynecol. Reprod. Biol.*, **11**, 319
7. Vanrell, J. A. and Balasch, J. (1983). Prolactin in the evaluation of luteal phase in infertility. *Fertil. Steril.*, **39**, 30
8. Schulz, K.-D., Geiger, W., del Pozo, E. and Künzig, H. J. (1978). Pattern of sexual steroids, prolactin and gonadotropic hormones during prolactin inhibition in normally cycling women. *Am. J. Obstet. Gynecol.*, **132**, 561
9. McNatty, K. P., Sawers, R. S. and McNeilly, A. S. (1974). A possible role for prolactin in control of steroid secretion by the human graafian follicle. *Nature*, **250**, 653
10. McNatty, K. P. (1979). Relationship between plasma prolactin and the endocrine microenvironment of the developing human antral follicle. *Fertil. Steril.*, **32**, 433
11. L'Hermite, M., Michaux-Duchêne, A. and Robyn, C. (1979). Tiapride-induced chronic hyperprolactinaemia: interference with the human menstrual cycle. *Acta Endocrinol. (Kbh)*, **92**, 214
12. L'Hermite, M., Denayer, P., Golstein, J., Virasoro, E., Vanhaelst, L., Copinschi, G. and Robyn, C. (1978). Acute endocrine profile of sulpiride in the human. *Clin. Endocrinol.*, **9**, 195
13. L'Hermite, M., McLeod, R. M. and Robyn, C. (1978). Effects of two substituted benzamides, tiapride and sultopride, on gonadotrophins and prolactin. *Acta Endocrinol. (Kbh)*, **98**, 29
14. McLeod, R. M. and Robyn, C. (1977). On the mechanism of increased prolactin secretion by sulpiride. *J. Endocrinol.*, **72**, 273
15. Portaleone, P., di Carlo, R., Crispino, A. and Genazzani, E. (1978). *Neurosci. Lett.*, **10**, 305
16. Chatani, F., Aono, T., Koike, K., Tasaka, K. and Kurachi, K. (1983). Effect of sulpiride induced hyperprolactinaemia on catecholamine turnover and LRH concentration in the medial basal hypothalamus of rats. *Acta Endocrinol. (Kbh)*, **102**, 321
17. L'Hermite, M., Vekemans, M., Caufriez, A., Martin-Comin, J., Delogne-Desnoeck, J. and Robyn, C. (In preparation) Interference with the human menstrual cycle by chronic sulpiride-induced hyperprolactinaemia
18. L'Hermite, M., Delogne-Desnoeck, J., Michaux-Duchêne, A. and Robyn, C. (1978). Alteration of feedback mechanism of estrogen on gonadotropin by sulpiride-induced hyperprolactinaemia. *J. Clin. Endocrinol. Metab.*, **47**, 1132
19. Andersen, A. N., Schiøler, V., Hertz, J. and Bennett, P. (1982). Effect of metoclopramide induced hyperprolactinaemia on the gonadotrophic response to oestradiol and LRH. *Acta Endocrinol. (Kbh)*, **100**, 1
20. Nakano, R. and Yagi, S. (1983). Feedback mechanism in sulpiride-induced hyperprolactinaemia. *Br. J. Obstet. Gynecol.*, **90**, 350
21. Buvat, J., Thomas, K., Racadot, A., Blacker, C., Buvat-Herbaut, M., Ferin, F. and Linquette, M. (1978). Changes in pituitary gonadotropins during the amenorrhoea-galactorrhoea syndrome due to sulpiride. *Clin. Endocrinol.*, **9**, 499

22. Huseman, C. A., Kugler, J. A. and Schneider, I. G. (1980). Mechanism of dopaminergic suppression of gonadotropin secretion in men. *J. Clin. Endocrinol. Metab.*, **51**, 209
23. Quigley, M. E., Sheehan, K. L., Casper, R. F. and Yen, S. S. C. (1980). Evidence for an increased opioid inhibition of luteinizing hormone secretion in hyperprolactinemic patients with pituitary microadenoma. *J. Clin. Endocrinol. Metab.*, **50**, 427
24. Leyendecker, G., Struve, T. and Plotz, E. J. (1980). Induction of ovulation with chronic intermittent (pulsatile) administration of LH-RH in women with hypothalamic and hyperprolactinemic amenorrhea. *Arch. Gynecol.*, **229**, 177
25. Aksel, S. (1980). Sporadic and recurrent luteal phase defects in cyclic women: comparison with normal cycles. *Fertil. Steril.*, **33**, 372
26. Kauppila, A., Leinonen, P., Vikko, R. and Ylöstalo, P. (1982). Metoclopramide-induced hyperprolactinemia impairs ovarian follicle maturation and corpus luteum function in women. *J. Clin. Endocrinol. Metab.*, **54**, 955
27. Coutts, J. R. T., Adam, A. H. and Fleming, R. (1982). The deficient luteal phase may represent an anovulatory cycle. *Clin. Endocrinol.*, **17**, 389
28. Cheung, C. Y. (1983). Prolactin suppresses luteinizing hormone secretion and pituitary responsiveness to luteinizing hormone-releasing hormone by a direct action at the anterior pituitary. *Endocrinology*, **113**, 632
29. Delvoye, P., Taubert, H.-D., Jürgensen, O., L'Hermite, M., Delogne, J. and Robyn, C. (1974). Evolution des gonadotrophines et de la progestérone sériques au cours d'une hyperprolactinémie induite par le sulpiride (Dogmatil) pendant la phase lutéale du cycle menstruel. *C.R. Acad. Sci. (Paris), Sér. D*, **279**, 1463
30. Robyn, C. (1980). Discussion. In L'Hermite, M. and Judd, S. J. (eds) *Advances in Prolactin.* p. 193 (Basel: Karger)
31. Coutts, J. R. T., Fleming, R., Craig, A., Barlow, D., England, P. and Macnaughton, M. C. (1980). Role of transient hyperprolactinaemia in the short luteal phase. In L'Hermite, M. and Judd, S. J. (eds) *Advances in Prolactin.* pp. 187–193 (Basel: Karger).
32. Ben-David, M. and Schenker, J. G. (1983). Transient hyperprolactinemia: a correctable cause of idiopathic female infertility. *J. Clin. Endocrinol. Metab.*, **57**, 442
33. Lenton, E. A., Brook, L. M., Sobowale, O. and Cooke, I. D. (1979). Prolactin concentrations in normal menstrual cycles and conception cycles. *Clin. Endocrinol.*, **10**, 383
34. Crosignani, P. G., Reschini, E., Lombroso, G. C., Arosio, M. and Peracchi, M. (1978). Comparison of placebo and bromocriptine in the treatment of patients with normoprolactinaemic amenorrhoea. *Br. J. Obstet. Gynecol.*, **85**, 773
35. Wright, C. S., Steele, S. J. and Jacobs, H. S. (1979). Value of bromocriptine in unexplained primary infertility: a double-blind controlled trial. *Br. Med. J.*, **1**, 1037
36. Coelingh-Bennink, H. J. T. and van der Steeg, H. J. (1983). Failure of bromocriptine to restore the menstrual cycle in normoprolactinemic post-pill amenorrhoea. *Fertil. Steril.*, **39**, 238
37. Maslar, I. A. and Riddick, D. H. (1979). Prolactin production by human endometrium during the normal menstrual cycle. *Am. J. Obstet. Gynecol.*, **135**, 751
38. Taga, M., Satoh, M., Minaguchi, H., Mizuno, M. and Sakamoto, S. (1982). Synthesis and secretion of prolactin in the decidualized human endometrium unassociated with pregnancy *in vitro. Endocrinol. Japon.*, **29**, 335
39. Daly, D. C., Maslar, I. A., Rosenberg, S. M., Tohan, N. and Riddick, D. H. (1981). Prolactin production by luteal phase defect endometrium. *Am. J. Obstet. Gynecol.*, **140**, 587

Discussion

Rothchild	I am grateful to hear the details of your findings and thoughts about the reasons for the disturbance of luteal and ovarian function in hyperprolactinaemia, because they agree so well with what I have thought myself, and I am also very happy that you ended with some remarks about prolactin and decidual tissue, and the possible rôle it might play, because I want to suggest that maybe one of the disturbances in the short luteal phase, or rather the infertility associated with the short luteal phase, may go back to this peculiarity of the human endometrium, when it is decidualized to make prolactin. The reason that I say this is that the effects of hCG on corpus luteum function in humans and monkeys do not duplicate exactly the effects of the implanting blastocyst, which suggests that there is something besides hCG, even though hCG is certainly important as one of the signals coming from the blastocyst that affects and, in particular, slows down the regression phase of the corpus luteum. But we are all very well aware of the fact that in non-pregnant women or non-pregnant monkeys treating with hCG does not reproduce the prolonged maintenance of progesterone secretion that we see in early pregnancy. It has to be something else, perhaps coming from the blastocyst which prolongs the secretion of progesterone in the presence of hCG. It is quite obvious from experimental work that prolonged treatment with hCG eventually induces regression of the corpus luteum, so something must prevent this. Whether it is prolactin from decidual tissue or something else coming from the decidual tissue associated with prolactin, I do not know. I would like to suggest that prolactin may be a signal of the efficiency and effectiveness of the decidual tissue to play this role of potentiating the effect of hCG or other hormones coming from the blastocyst that prolong the secretion of the corpus luteum until eventually progesterone secretion by the placenta becomes dominant and maintains the pregnancy. And this may be one of the places where infertility comes in because of a breakdown of this rôle of decidual tissue.
Wentz	Professor Rothchild, what you have said about hCG not being able to maintain the corpus luteum function is true for the experiments that I know have been performed in the human in which hCG has been administered on a daily or every-other-daily basis using 5000 or 10 000 IU. However, to my knowledge, the correct experiment has not been performed, and that is to mimic what is happening in early pregnancy with respect to hCG measurements in the peripheral circulation. One has to attempt a doubling every other 2 days of hCG administration. If this were to be done – and it has been attempted only for 10 days because the doses of hCG got so high that it was simply impossible to administer them. But if this were done, would you predict whether perhaps the corpus luteum might respond, whereas it does not when the doses are maintained at a lower level?
Rothchild	I do not think it would, because the corpus luteum in the human pregnancy

57

responds up to about the fifth or sixth week *post ovulationem*, and then, if one follows 17α-OH-progesterone as an indication of corpus luteum function, there is a very slow regression that continues for the rest of pregnancy, in spite of the fact that hCG is present. So, there is something about the effect of hCG itself, even in high doses, which does not allow the corpus luteum to respond continuously. This piece of evidence is almost indicative that some other factors are involved in the response of the corpus luteum to hCG.

Bettendorf   I remember some experiments by Kaiser who did what you mentioned, i.e. doubling the dose of hCG comparably to the early pregnancy, and he showed that it is possible to stimulate luteal function up to 4–6 weeks (Kaiser R. and Geiger W.: *Acta Endocrinol.* **67** (1971), 331).

Koninckx   It has repeatedly been shown that there is no testosterone elevation in cycles with a short luteal phase, whereas in the normal cycle you have a small but significant elevation of testosterone at the time of the LH-peak. Could you comment on that; in particular whether this might be a prolactin effect?

L'Hermite   We did not measure testosterone in our experiments. This testosterone increase has been suggested to be involved in FSH release at midcycle, and it has been reported that the FSH peak may be missing in the short luteal phase cycle.

Schneider   You did not comment too much on interference by opioides with prolactin. You are aware of the work of Yen and co-workers who infused nalaxone during the luteal phase of normally menstruating women, and in this way increased the frequency of LH-pulsatility. Similarly, del Pozo and co-workers infused met-enkephalin into women on day 5 or day 7 of a normal menstrual cycle, and in this way abolished LH-pulsatility. By adding naloxone they could re-establish LH-pulsatility. This seems to indicate that it is not prolactin itself, but it is the opioides acting at the level of the hypothalamus by varying the frequency of LH-release rather than the amplitude.

You also mentioned an impairment of the positive feedback as a possible cause of interference with hypothalamic function. This has been very much disputed by Knobil and his associates, and all those who have tried to adapt the results of experiments in the monkey to the human female. It has been shown by Ferin and his group that in the follicular phase of the female rhesus monkey there is a low amplitude and a high frequency of LH-RH pulsatility. In the castrated monkey the frequency remains the same but the amplitude is increased. This indicates that estrogens modulate the amplitude of LH-RH secretion into the portal blood rather than the frequency, as opioides seem to do.

L'Hermite   I have said indeed that it was probably the pulsatility of GnRH-release which is disturbed, and you have been one of the first to show this in hyperprolactinaemic patients. Opioides certainly provide one of the mechanisms by which LH-pulsatility can be modified.

As far as the positive feedback of estradiol is concerned, I agree that this has been a somewhat disputed issue, although it has regularly been reported. It has usually been disputed when higher doses of estrogens have been given than probably required. As a consequence, it seems to be a matter of threshold.

Schneider   Did you mean to say that prolactin is just a marker rather than something having a direct effect?

L'Hermite   I quite agree that an elevated prolactin level is probably only a reflection of some other process, and I suggested this for transient or unapparent hyperprolactinaemia, although I am still convinced that a high prolactin level is causative when it is permanent even though it is the result of some other perturbation.

Dericks-Tan   As prolactin rises nocturnally, could it be expected that the chance for suffering from anovulatory disturbances rises in women with the length of the sleep-period?

L'Hermite
Such a correlation has indeed been suggested, and Bohnet, for example, has demonstrated that there is a relationship between the nocturnal prolactin surge and the magnitude of the prolactin response to metoclopramide. But I personally await clinical evidence that it really has an effect.

Rothchild
I cannot remember in which paper we reported that, but a suppression of the nocturnal rise of prolactin to normal levels in women with inadequate luteal phase and infertility had no effect whatsoever on the endometrial discrepancy, i.e. the discrepancy between the endometrial change and the progesterone pattern. I doubt if the nocturnal prolactin surge has very much of an influence.

Braendle
I would like to comment on decidual prolactin production since it has been speculated that it might have something to do with ovarian function. We have data on a hypophysectomized patient without measurable levels of prolactin who conceived during treatment with hMG/hCG. Prolactin remained unmeasurable throughout her pregnancy with the exception of one value obtained in the 18th week. At the time of delivery amniotic fluid was obtained and was found to contain 500 ng/ml. Moreover, for a short time following delivery we were also able to demonstrate prolactin in the blood of the patient.

5
Endometrial defect as morphological evidence of the inadequate luteal phase

GISELA DALLENBACH-HELLWEG

Since normal implantation of a fertilized ovum depends on a precise physiological balance between numerous factors of a structural and functional nature, subtle variations may suffice to cause infertility. Almost all functional disturbances involved in the genesis of the inadequate luteal phase result in morphological changes in the endometrium which represents the most important end-station for the implanting blastocyst. Serum hormone levels, even when measured with modern methods, fluctuate depending upon various biorhythms, resulting for example in a wide range of normal progesterone values for each day of the cycle. In addition, the histological finding of glandular stromal disparity cannot be determined by progesterone measurements. The most reliable method for diagnosing a functional disturbance of the endometrium therefore remains the histological study, and dating of a properly taken and accurately timed biopsy which serves as a bioassay measuring the hormone at the tissue level[1-3]. The biopsy also provides tissue for progesterone receptor studies which may help explain proliferating or deficiently secreting endometrium with elevated progesterone levels. What is important is selecting the proper time to perform a curettage, that is at the end of a menstrual cycle, shortly before bleeding begins.

The inadequate luteal phase is associated with a progesterone deficiency. The stimulatory effect of progesterone on the endometrium becomes deficient when the hormonal balance shifts in favour of estrogen. The progesterone deficiency can be absolute, when in the presence of an insufficient corpus luteum the production or secretion of progesterone is suppressed, or relative when hyperestrogenism develops. An *absolute progesterone deficiency* may occur after normal ovulation, if the corpus luteum fails to develop normally or regresses too quickly because of a central or ovarian defect such as inadequate luteinization of the granulosa cells because the LH peak is too low or too short-lasting; suppression of progesterone release by evelated prolactin levels[4], or inability of the oocytes to induce follicular development[5]. A *relative progesterone deficiency* may follow a preceding follicular persistency with delayed ovulation. The associated secretory phase is of normal length or may show an early breakdown of the endometrium. In other instances the corpus luteum insufficiency is preceded by impaired follicular development with inadequate stimulation of the granulosa cells which may be caused by insufficient FSH secretion in the early follicular phase. In these instances progesterone cannot fully act on the deficiently proliferated endometrium. In most of these conditions the plasma progesterone concentrations during the luteal phase are low[6-8]. In rare instances a defect of progesterone receptors in the endometrium may be the cause for a relative progesterone deficiency in the presence of a normal functioning corpus luteum ('pseudo-corpus luteum insufficiency')[9].

According to the degree of insufficiency, which may have central or ovarian causes, the resulting deficiency of the secretory phase varies, and infertility may come about by failure of the blastocyst to implant or by early unrecognized abortion. Since the result of treatment for this type of infertility depends on the accuracy of its diagnosis, a precise differentiation between the various patterns of the deficient secretory phase seems of paramount importance (Table 5.1).

Just as the type and cause of disturbance or interference in the function of the corpus luteum may vary, so may the histological picture of the resultant deficient secretory phase fluctuate[10].

The deficient secretory phase with dissociated delay, which is the most frequently encountered variety, shows widely spaced, poorly convoluted glands, a variation in the development of glands and stroma from region to region, and a dissociation of development between glands and their surrounding stroma. Adjacent to fairly normal secretory glands which roughly correspond with the proper day of the cycle, one may see other glands which are poorly developed with basal vacuoles and small rounded nuclei in low, functionally inactive, epithelial cells. Other glands, however, may still be in a state of proliferation and contain elongated nuclei with dense chromatin in a non-functioning, hormonally unresponsive epithelium (Figure 5.1). The variation in glandular differentiation results from decreased progesterone levels. Only those portions close to the blood supply receive enough progesterone to react properly. The regions with the lowest hormone concentrations show the poorest differentiation of their glandular cells, and the lowest glycogen content, whereas acid mucopolysaccharides may still be found. Accordingly, the glandular epithelium contains variably diminished amounts of glycogen, mucopolysaccharides, proteins and acid phosphatases[11]. The activity of the alkaline phosphatase is often increased[12, 13]. Electron-microscopically the granules of glycogen, the mitochondria and the intranucleolar channel system of the glandular cells are reduced in size and number[14, 15]. The concentrations of estrogen receptors in the nucleus and cytoplasm are lower than in the normal secretory phase. The concentrations of progesterone receptors correspond to the low values of the delayed secretory phase[16]. The prolactin production by endometrial explants *in vitro* correlates with the degree of predecidual transformation of the stroma and accordingly is diminished as compared with normal secretory phase endometrium[17]. The stroma may be poorly differentiated and focally oedematous, in other areas large-celled, even with predecidual change and

Table 5.1 Causes of the inadequate luteal phase

	Proliferative phase	Ovulation	Length of secretory phase	Corpus luteum	Gonadotropin	Cause
Co-ordinated apparent delay	Prolonged and irregular	Delayed	Normal or early breakdown	Normal or early regression	Late LH peak	Central defect in LH stimulation, e.g. hyperprolactinaemia
Co-ordinated true delay	Shortened and deficient	Too early	Short or normal	Deficient	Low FSH	(1) Central defect: inadequate stimulation of granulosa cells
	Normal length and deficient	At proper time	Short or normal	Normal or slightly deficient		(2) Ovarian defect: impaired follicular development
	Normal		Normal	Normal	Normal	Endometrial progesterone receptor defect
Dissociated delay	Normal	At proper time	Short or normal	Deficient	Low or short-lasting LH peak	Central defect: (a) inadequate luteinization of granulosa cells; (b) suppression of progesterone release by hyperprolactinaemia
				Normal	Normal	Endometrial progesterone receptor defect

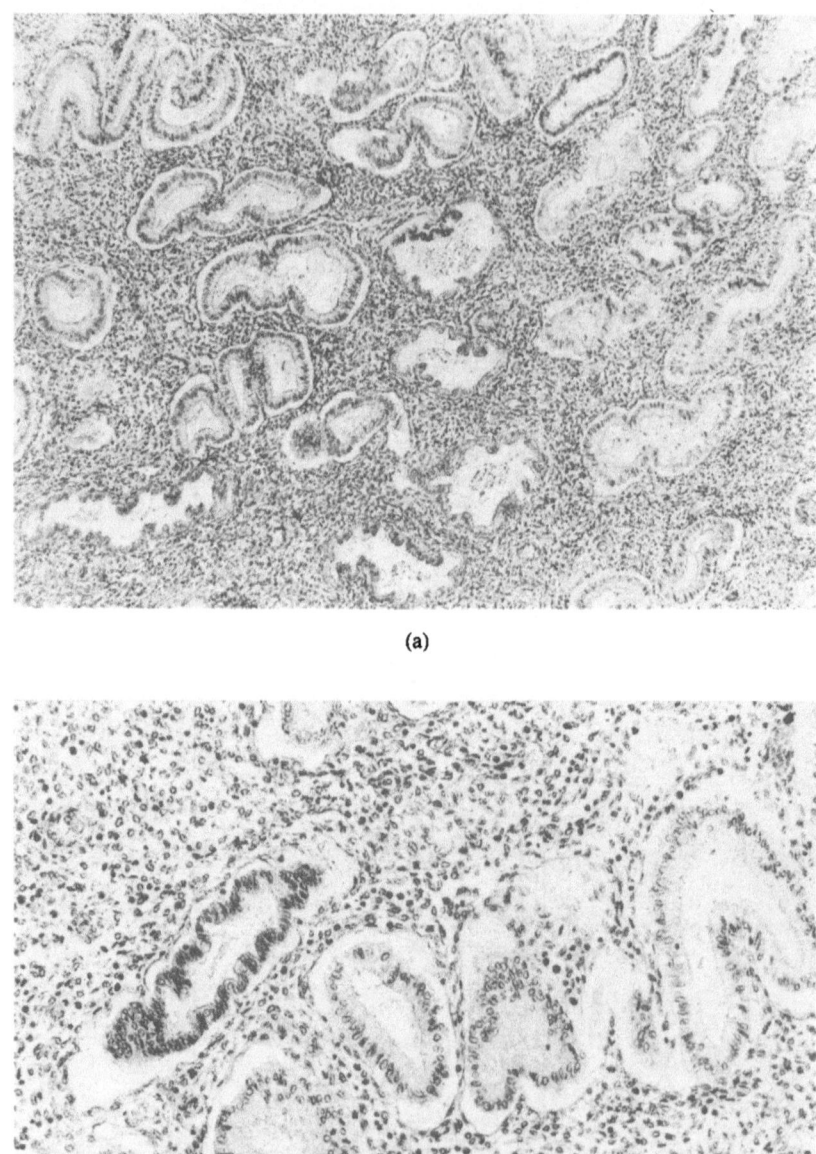

(a)

(b)

Figure 5.1 Deficient secretory phase with dissociated delay of glands and stroma; 27th day of a menstrual cycle. Haematoxylin and eosin stain. Magnification (a) ×50, (b) ×125

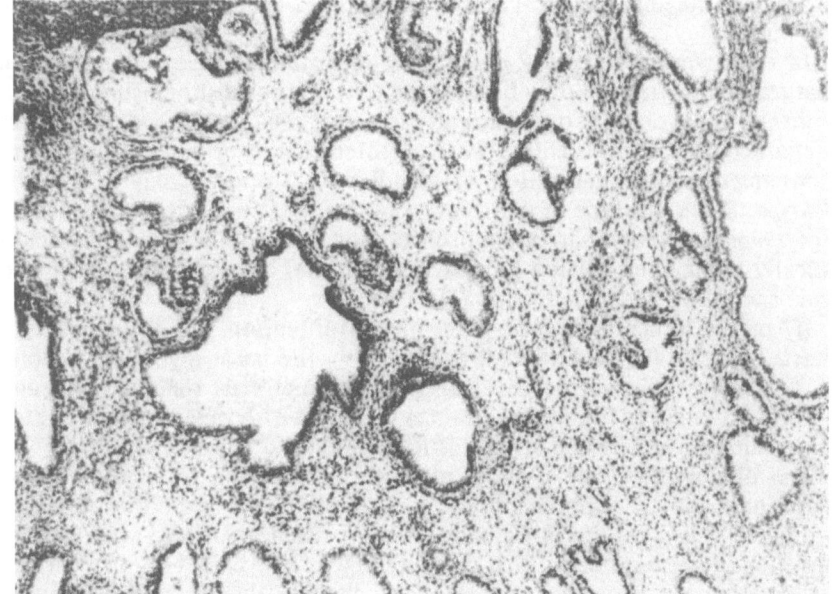

Figure 5.2 Deficient secretory phase with co-ordinated apparent delay of maturation. Partly dilated glands in beginning secretion; 26th day of a menstrual cycle. Haematoxylin and eosin stain. Magnification ×40

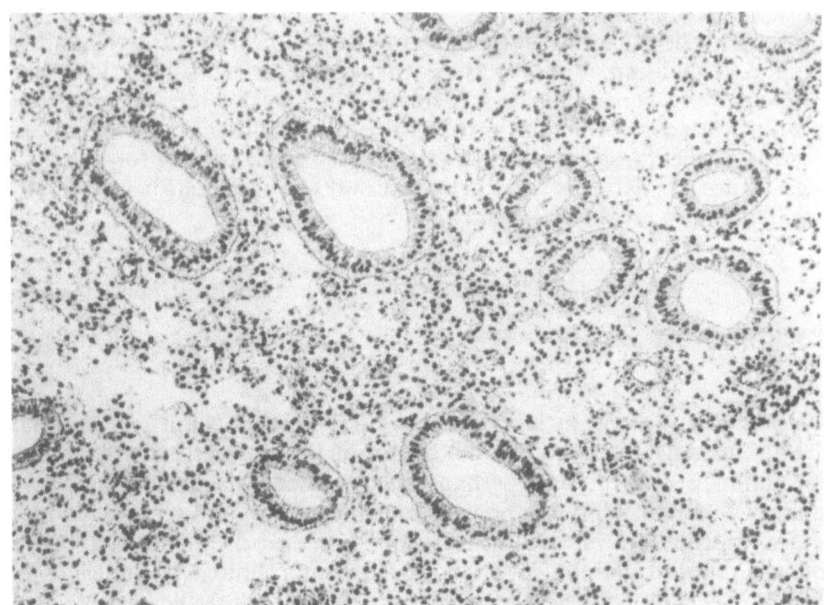

Figure 5.3 Deficient secretory phase with co-ordinated true delay in differentiation. Narrow straight glands in beginning secretion on the 25th day of a cycle. Haematoxylin and eosin stain. Magnification ×125

local small haemorrhages. The spiral arterioles remain small and under-developed.

In the *deficient secretory phase with co-ordinated delay*, this delay in maturation is often the only histological criterion for distinguishing it from a normal luteal phase. To find an early secretory phase at the end of the cycle is characteristic for this entity, which is often caused by delayed ovulation. Consequently, the maturation of glands and stroma is only *apparently delayed*. Since this type of deficient secretory phase was often preceded by a persistent follicle with irregular proliferation, some of the glands character-istically retain their dilated lumina. The stromal cells are fairly large and wide-spaced by oedema (Figure 5.2).

If, on the other hand, the preceding proliferation was insufficient or shortened, the glands are small and narrow, the basal glycogen vacuoles hardly reach their normal size, and the stromal cells remain small and undifferentiated. In these rare instances we have a *truly delayed* co-ordinated maturation of glands and stroma (Figure 5.3).

The dissociated delay is most often the result of a true progesterone deficiency due to suppression of its production or secretion. The co-ordinated delay, on the other hand, is most often associated with normal secretion of progesterone which is counteracted by an excess of estrogen, for instance from a preceding persistent follicle. In other cases progesterone cannot fully act because of a preceding deficient proliferation with under-development of glands and stroma.

Twenty-five per cent of all the deficient secretory phases are abnormally short, and at times last only 8 days[18]. The shedding of the endometrium starts prematurely because the levels of progesterone decline earlier than they should. In addition, bleeding is protracted; it starts in areas with well-differentiated stromal cells and involves other areas later. The menstrual shedding with correct dissolution of stromal and glandular elements can take place only when progesterone has acted on the endometrium for at least 10 days. Hence, the deficient secretory phase may also terminate in pathological bleeding due to estrogen withdrawal.

CONCLUSION

The pathologist serves as an important guide in the diagnosis of the cause of infertility, helping to direct the course of the clinician's investigations. The ultimate refined, and perhaps subclassified, diagnosis remains the clinician's responsibility, as he calls on other techniques to provide more precise information. These same techniques, on the other hand, receive their control, support and confirmation from the morphological studies of the pathologist. Here, in the diagnosis and treatment of infertile patients, as in medicine in general, it is only through an indispensable close co-operation between clinician and pathologist that optimal care of the patient can be provided.

References

1. Jones, G. S., Aksel, S. and Wentz, A. C. (1974). Serum progesterone values in the luteal phase defects: effects of chorionic gonadotropin. *Obstet. Gynecol.*, **44**, 26
2. Annos, T., Thompson, I. E. and Taymor, M. L. (1980). Luteal phase deficiency and infertility: difficulties encountered in diagnosis and treatment. *Obstet. Gynecol.*, **55**, 705
3. Rosenfeld, D. L., Chodow, S. and Bronson, R. A. (1980). Diagnosis of luteal phase inadequacy. *Obstet. Gynecol.*, **56**, 193
4. Taubert, H.-D. (1978). Luteal phase insufficiency. In Keller, P. J. (ed.) *Contrib. Gynecol. Obstet.* vol. 4, pp. 78–113. (Basel: S. Karger)
5. Fox, H. and Buckley, C. H. (1982). Pathologic factors involved in infertility. In Blaustein, A. (ed.) *A Pathology of the Female Genital Tract.* pp. 828–837. (New York, Heidelberg, Berlin: Springer-Verlag)
6. Moszkowski, E., Woodruff, J. D. and Jones, G. E. S. (1962). The inadequate luteal phase. *Am. J. Obstet. Gynecol.*, **83**, 363
7. Abraham, G. E., Maroulis, G. B. and Marshall, J. R. (1974). Evaluation of ovulation and corpus luteum function using measurements of plasma progesterone. *Obstet. Gynecol.*, **44**, 522
8. Radwanska, E. and Swyer, G. I. M. (1974). Plasma progesterone estimation in infertile women and in women under treatment with clomiphene and chorionic gonadotropins. *J. Obstet. Br. Commonw.*, **81**, 107
9. Keller, D. W., Wiest, W. G., Askin, F. B., Johnson, L. W. and Strickler, R. C. (1979). Pseudocorpus luteum insufficiency: a local defect of progesterone action on endometrial tissue. *J. Clin. Endocrinol. Metab.*, **48**, 127
10. Gigon, U., Herzer, H., Stamm, O. and Zarro, D. (1970). Endometriumveränderungen und luteotrope Sekretionsanomalien bei Gelbkörperinsuffizienz. *Z. Geburtschilfe Gynäkol.*, **173**, 304
11. Hughes, E. C., Jacobs, R. D. and Rubulis, A. (1964). Effect of treatment for sterility and abortion upon the carbohydrate pathways of the endometrium. *Am. J. Obstet. Gynecol.*, **89**, 59
12. Noyes, R. W. (1959). The underdeveloped secretory endometrium. *Am. J. Obstet. Gynecol.*, **77**, 929
13. Schmidt-Mathiessen, H. (1965). Die dysfunktionelle uterine Blutung. Histochemie und Mechanismus. *Gynaecologia* (Basel), **160**, 197
14. Ancla, M., de Brux, J., Musset, R. and Bret, J. A. (1967). Etude au microscope électronique de l'endomètre humain dans différentes conditions d'équilibre hormonal. *Arch. Pathol.*, **15**, 136
15. Gore, B. Z. and Gordon, M. (1974). Fine structure of epithelial cell of secretory endometrium in unexplained primary infertility. *Fertil. Steril.*, **25**, 103
16. Levy, C., Robel, P., Gautray, J. P., De Brux, J., Verma, U., Descomps, B., Baulieu, E. E. and Eychenne, B. (1980). Estradiol and progesterone receptors in human endometrium: Normal and abnormal menstrual cycles and early pregnancy. *Am. J. Obstet. Gynecol.*, **136**, 646
17. Daly, C. D., Maslar, I. A., Rosenberg, S. M., Tohan, N. and Riddick, D. H. (1981). Prolactin production by luteal phase defect endometrium. *Am. J. Obstet. Gynecol.*, **140**, 587
18. Buxton, C. L. (1950). The atypical secretory phase. In Engle, E. T. (ed.) *Menstruation and its Disorders.* p. 270. (Springfield, Ill.: Charles C. Thomas)

Discussion

Schneider	You said that you would be able to differentiate between ovulation and anovulation, and even to recognize the luteinized unruptured follicle syndrome. Do you prefer biopsies to other diagnostic tools, e.g. to progesterone measurements?
Dallenbach-Hellweg	I believe I can differentiate ovulation from anovulation, because the appearance of the glandular nuclei, the size of the basal vacuoles, the shape of the glands and the stromal cells look quite different if the persistent follicle is only partly luteinized.
Schneider	Biologically speaking, to look at the target organ always makes more sense than to look at the substrate. But I cannot imagine that this is really possible.
Dallenbach-Hellweg	The endometrium reacts very sensitively to any hormonal stimulus. If you obtain a secretory endometrium you can judge what the proliferative phase was like. It is a very precise method of diagnosing a functional disturbance.
Insler	Would you be able to diagnose on a biopsy the presence of a few luteinized follicles, resulting in reversing the estrogen/progesterone ratio?
Dallenbach-Hellweg	I think, when I have the precise day of the cycle and some other parameters, I could do it.
Rothchild	I am very curious about the remark concerning that woman who ovulated regularly on hMG but remained amenorrhoeic. How different is the endometrium histologically from that of a woman who menstruates regularly?
Dallenbach-Hellweg	It is a very rare case, but you can see all degrees between this extreme and normal menstruation, because the endometrium sheds only to a certain degree. Some patients shed only about the first millimetre and all the remaining functionalis and basalis is regenerated and re-incorporated into the next menstrual cycle. In the newly proliferating endometrium you can see regenerating glands from the previous cycle that had been secreting. This is precisely what you see in patients who have no menstruation.
Wentz	The only time I have ever seen that this happened, is in a condition that we call Asherman's syndrome or endometrial sclerosis. However, following many anovulatory biphasic temperature cycles that are non-bleeding, I have never seen what you described and I found it fascinating to hear you describe it.
Dallenbach-Hellweg	The picture of dissociated delay of maturation, i.e. the dissociated deficient secretory phase, shows focally secreting glands in the close neighbourhood of cells which are still proliferating, and this is mostly due to a too low progesterone level which only reaches those portions of the endometrium close to the blood supply. It is no individual disposition and you can see it frequently, particularly in the climacteric woman with corpus luteum deficiencies, but also in younger infertile patients.
Dericks-Tan	Perez *et al.* (*Fertil. Steril.*, **35**, (1981), 423) demonstrated that endometrial histological findings do not in all instances reflect ovarian function. They

68

found in some cases a proliferated endometrium in the presence of a corpus luteum and in others no corpus luteum but a secretory endometrium.

Dallenbach-Hellweg I mentioned that you may have a functioning corpus luteum and still an atrophic or proliferating endometrium in cases of a progesterone receptor defect. But studying large series, there is a good correlation between corpus luteum and endometrium in over 80%.

Wentz The definition of luteal phase inadequacy that we have used for many years has indeed been based on the target organ, the endometrium. If we take the endometrial biopsy as close as possible to the anticipated menses, then an expected pattern will be seen 1 or 2 days before the expected menses. One can take the biopsy based perhaps on the temperature chart, perhaps on the history of regular menses, or perhaps one might simply rub a crystal ball. I will show you three cases of biopsies taken as close as possible to the expected menses. The first shows an endometrium which fulfilled the criteria for day 25/26. This individual had menses 2 days later and this biopsy was, therefore, called in-phase. The second biopsy shows a pattern identical to the first. This individual had the menses about 6 hours after this biopsy was taken and, therefore, by our way of definition, it would be read as 2–3 days out-of-phase and suggestive of luteal phase inadequacy. The third biopsy again shows an identical pattern. It is in a patient who did not get menses and the reason, of course, was that she was pregnant. The point is that the endometrial biopsy material may be identical in three diverse situations. Therefore, we have to be very careful with using endometrial biopsy evidence and it should be correlated with what happens during the cycle.

Koninckx The question is whether biopsy could be harmful for implantation. At this moment we have 37 endometrium biopsies taken during the cycle of conception. All the datings were the 19th day or later in the cycle, and a biopsy taken in the early luteal phase should be harmful for implantation.

Dallenbach-Hellweg The early luteal phase is not the right time to take an endometrial biopsy. It should be taken as close to the expected menstruation as possible; sometimes you may even take it when menstruation had already started. It is still possible to diagnose infertility on this biopsy, while in the early luteal phase it is very difficult because you really do not know how the luteal phase is going to develop.

Rothchild I think that is a beautiful demonstration of the problems of histological diagnosis. Dr Wentz has shown that the patient can get pregnant with an endometrium that does not seem to be at the right stage of development for that part of the cycle. While in the rat the endometrium has to undergo a very precise change in a very precise time after ovulation, I think that the human may be one among several types of mammals in which there is no very strict relationship between the degree of development and the time the blastocyst implants. And I wonder whether we should not look for other things, e.g. prolactin and the production of prolactin by human decidual tissue. It may be a very important factor in determining whether pregnancy starts or does not start, or does start and not continue.

69

6
Ultrastructural and endocrine studies of endometrial biopsies during the inadequate luteal phase

M. R. KÖHLER, K.-W. SCHWEPPE, J. P. HANKER,
H. THEMANN AND H. P. G. SCHNEIDER

MATERIAL AND METHODS

Twelve female outpatients, who presented with primary sterility and the syndrome of a defective luteal phase, were selected for this study. A defective luteal phase was defined as a short ($\leqslant 10$ days) hyperthermic phase of the basal body temperature associated in most instances with an inadequate ($\leqslant 60$ nmol/l) mid-luteal (day 22) progesterone level. Other endocrine disorders – such as diabetes mellitus, adrenal or thyroid dysfunction – had been ruled out prior to this investigation. All patients were normoprolactinaemic – as assessed by metoclopramide tests – and their body weights were within the normal limits. The study was performed during an untreated control cycle. Uterine biopsies were taken without anaesthesia under hysteroscopic control from different areas of the fundus endometrium on day 12 and 22 from two patients and with biopsy forceps from the uterine fundus on day 12 and 22 in 10 patients.

The samples were fixed immediately in a solution of 3% glutaraldehyde, pH 7.2 at 4 °C for 2 h. After being cut into 1 mm^3 pieces the tissue was post-fixed in 1.33% osmium tetroxide for 60 min and dehydrated with increasing concentrations of ethanol. Embedding was performed in three steps over a period of 24 h in Epon 812. Sections of approximately 1 μm thickness were cut with the LKB ultramicrotome, stained with toluidine blue in 1% borax, pH 12, and examined under the light microscope for orientation. After trimming of selected areas thin sections were cut and mounted on uncoated 300-mesh copper grids. The post-staining was performed with alcoholic uranyl acetate and lead nitrate, and sections were examined with the Philips EM 301.

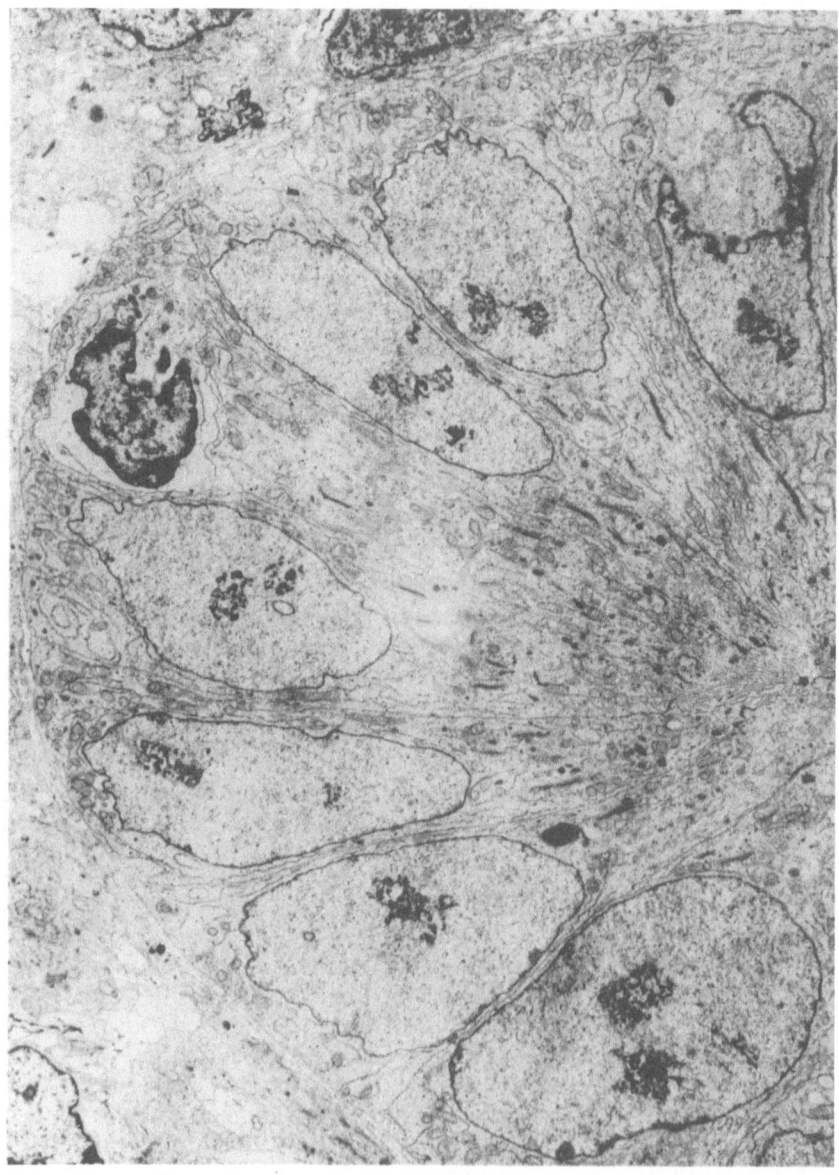

Figure 6.1 Endometrium at day 12 of a CLI cycle showing typical proliferating epithelial cells (IA), which correlate with the mid-proliferative phase of a normal cycle ($\times 5320$)

RESULTS

Late proliferative phase

The ultrastructural features of the endometrium of the late proliferative phase (day 12) of patients with corpus luteum inadequacy (CLI) are characterized by inadequate development of the glandular epithelium and by the appearance of different cell types in the same gland. The uterine mucosa of three patients shows epithelial cells, which are delayed in growth and cytoplasmic differentiation in comparison to late proliferative endometrium of a normal menstrual cycle (group IA; Figure 6.1). The volume of the cells is reduced and numerous S-folds of the intercellular membranes can be observed reaching the supranuclear part of the cells. The high cylindrical epithelium tapers toward the lumen. The apical membranes form moderate cytoplasmic protrusions with only moderately developed microvilli. The nuclei are elongated and irregularly shaped in a basal position. The karyoplasm is granular, mostly euchromatic with one or two nucleoli. The rough endoplasmic reticulum (rER) is well developed in contrast to the poorly developed smooth ER. In the apical and basal portion of the cells mitochondria are frequently seen. They are small and round or oval and are almost without intramitochondrial granules. Few small Golgi complexes can be found in the cytoplasm, sometimes forming a typical half-moon structure around the apical part of the nucleus. Glycogen is very sparsely distributed, even in the basal part of the cells. In the supranuclear cytoplasm osmiophilic dense bodies can be found, while multivesicular bodies are rare. The lumina of the glands are narrow, and only little cytoplasmic material is visible in the fine dispersed luminal substance.

The biopsies of nine patients represent a heterogeneous morphology in different areas of the same gland (group II A,B,C: Figure 6.2). Differences can be demonstrated with respect to electron density, cytoplasmic differentiation, and structures of the organelles. The predominant cell type – characterized as typical for CLI-endometrium (group IIA) – is highly cylindrical with an irregular basal lamina. The intercellular membranes show many S-folds up to the apical part of the cells, and in the basal parts the intercellular distances can be widened. The apical membrane is almost flat, sometimes interrupted by small, cylindrical protrusions or concave invaginations with a suggestion of missing cytoplasmic material. The microvilli appear in large numbers, and are highly developed, long and small, and thickened on top of the protrusions. The nucleus is irregularly shaped, round or elongated with a basal position. The karyoplasm contains some heterochromatic spots, especially in the border areas. One or two nucleoli can be found. The rER forms a dense network of folded membranes mostly in the subnuclear areas. Proliferation of four or five granular membranes can be observed in the supranuclear cytoplasm of some cells, resembling the structures of annulate lamellae. Mitochondria are frequent, small in size, round or longitudinal-shaped with only few cristae. The Golgi complexes are composed of three stretched apparatuses, formed by four or five dictyosomes, surrounded by some small vesicles. Glycogen is distributed as spots, which form very rarely

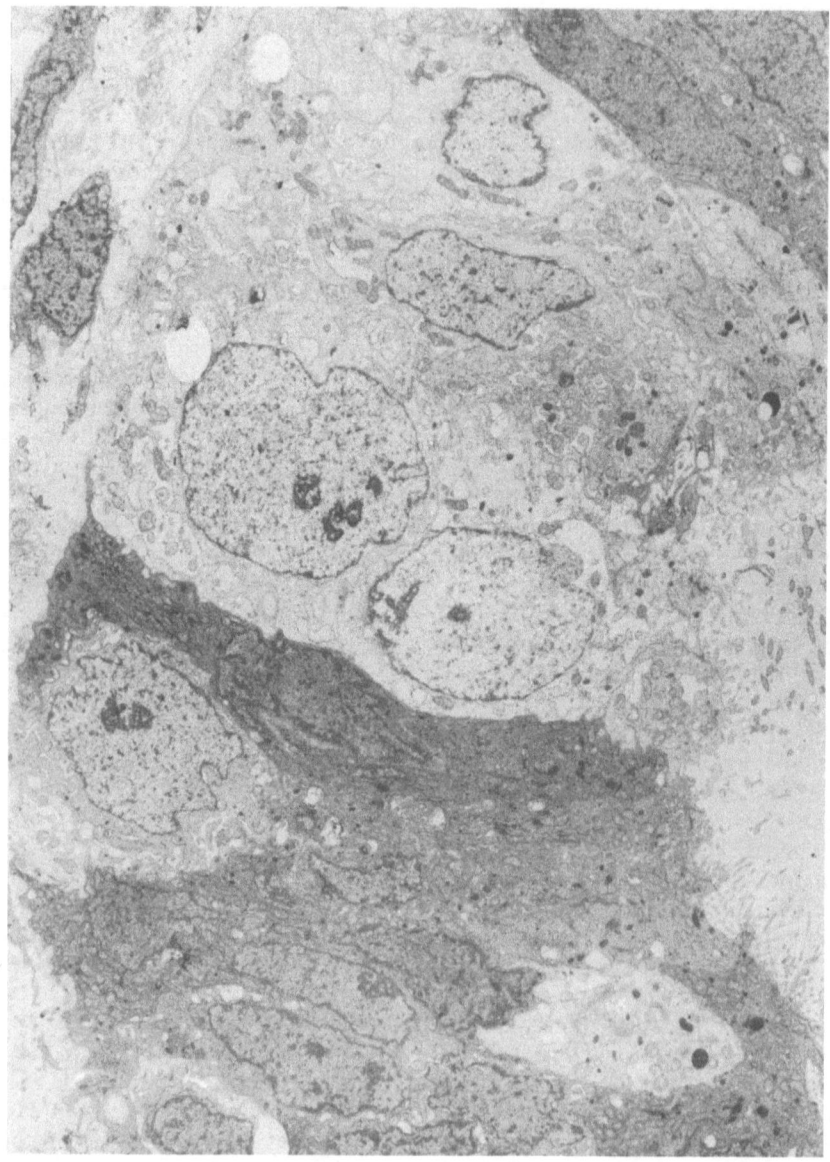

Figure 6.2 Endometrium at day 12 of a CLI cycle showing morphological variations of different cell types. Typical epithelial cells (group IIA) in the lower half; electron-light cells with signs of degeneration (group IIB) and in the right upper corner an electron-dense cell (group IIC) (×4620)

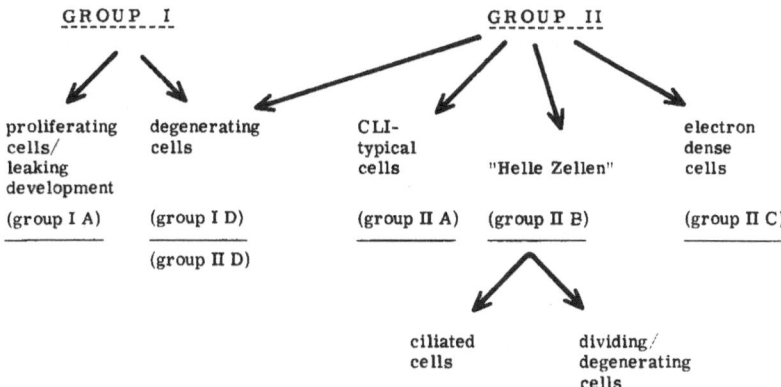

Figure 6.3 Cell types of the uterine mucosa in the late proliferating phase (day 12)

confluenting patches. In between this type of epithelium some cells show an electron-light karyoplasm and cytoplasm (group IIB). Some of them are ciliated cells, which belong to the group of 'Helle Zellen' because of their reduced content of ribosomes and organelles. These cells are found alone or in clusters, and are surrounded by epithelial cells with higher electron density. The nuclear–cytoplasmic ratio increases, and the regularly shaped nucleus adapts to the shape of the cell. The karyoplasm seems to be void of chromatic material. Small granules – similar to nucleolar ribosomes – can be found, producing a more electron-dense karyoplasm when they appear in clusters. Nucleoli are mostly missing, and the nuclear envelope is widened and connected to a blown-up rER. Glycogen cannot be observed. The apical membrane is nearly flat, with luminal openings in some areas, where organelles and cytoplasmic material are released, suggesting merocrine secretion.

Some cells impress because of their heterochromatic nucleus and increased content of organelles in an electron-dense cytoplasm (dark cells; group IIC; Figure 6.4) as a result of many ribosomes. Some cells show an interrupted nuclear envelope, and karyoplasm and cytoplasm seem mixed. Some of these cells contain more homogeneously distributed glycogen. In addition, ciliated cells are found, which show the typical ultrastructural features. Other areas of the same biopsies demonstrate different degrees of degeneration and disorganization of the lining epithelium (group ID and IID; Figure 6.6) as demonstrated by the different cell types of the uterine mucosa in the late proliferative phase of CLI patients.

To demonstrate the different cell types of the uterine mucosa of day 12 of CLI patients a schematic overview is given in Figure 6.3.

Mid-secretory phase (day 8 after ovulation):

All biopsies taken on day 8 after ovulation are characterized by an insufficient secretory transformation of the uterine mucosa. The glandular epithelial cells can be divided in two groups:

75

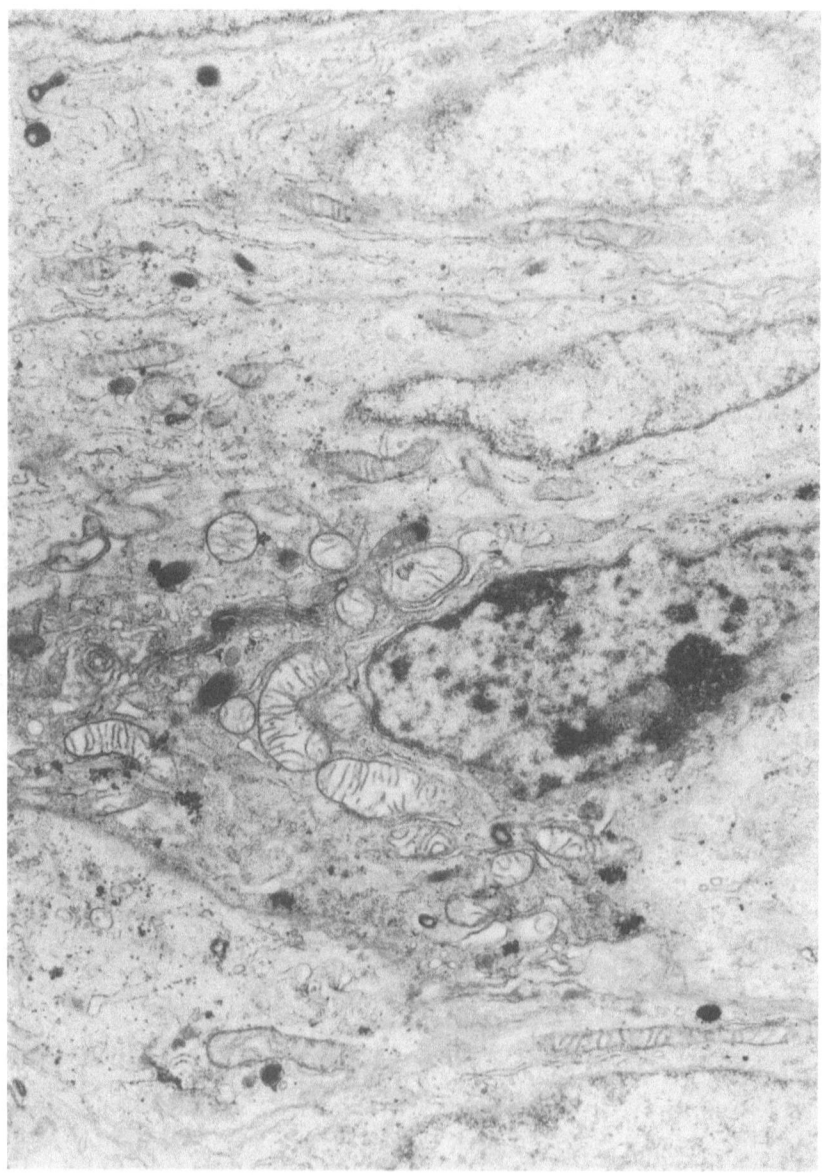

Figure 6.4 Glandular epithelial cell (group IIC) of the uterine mucosa at day 12 of a CLI cycle. An electron-dense cell with swollen mitochondria and many free ribosomes is surrounded by typical proliferating cells (group IIA) (×16 720)

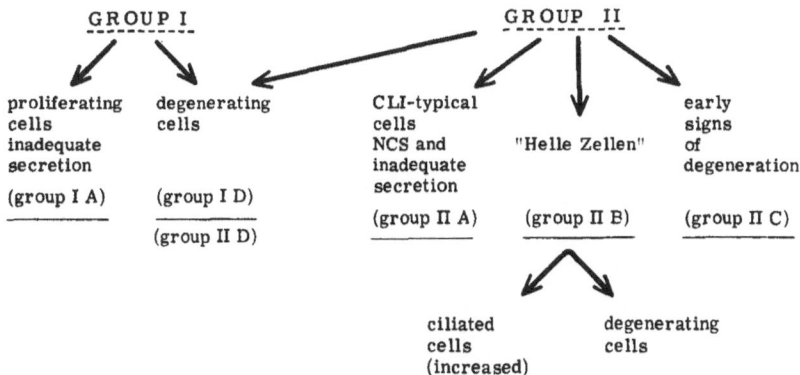

Figure 6.5 All types of the uterine mucosa of a CLI cycle (day 22)

(1) cells which show still the ultrastructural features of the late proliferative phase, without characteristic signs of the postovulatory phase such as the nuclear channel system (NCS) – except one case – giant mitochondria and large patches of confluent glycogen;

(2) cells which are inhomogeneously differentiated; some showing secretory transformations and the development of a NCS.

The endometrium of the three patients, which was described as delayed in the biopsies on day 12, on day 8 after ovulation still show signs of proliferation without typical secretory changes (group IA; Figure 6.7). The basal lamina is flat and the shape of the epithelium is highly prismatic. Well-developed apical protrusions contain some glycogen, small vesicles, and small tubuli of smooth ER. The regular configurated nucleus is in mid-position, elongated, and contains euchromatic karyoplasm with one nucleolus in peripheral position. Free ribosomes, polysomes, and rER are well-developed while mitochondria remain small and elongated. In the subnuclear area a small amount of glycogen is observed forming granular β-particles, which are often clustered. The lumen of the glands contains an increased amount of secretory products. Other areas of these biopsies show a cylindrical epithelium with flattened apical membranes, featuring highly developed microvilli. The nuclei are irregularly shaped with more heterochromatic karyoplasm. The supranuclear part of the cells is electron-light. Some mitosis can be observed. The number of ciliated cells has increased.

The biopsies of the remaining nine patients contain a mixture of different cell types, as already described on day 12 of the cycle (group IIA,B,C; Figure 6.8). The predominant cell type – characterized as typical for CLI-endometrium (group IIA) has undergone insufficient secretory changes, but in some of these cells a NCS was found. The shape is moderately prismatic and the apical cytoplasmic protrusions are prominent. The nuclei lie in midposition, and contain some condensed spots of chromatin and nucleolar ribosomes. Mostly, the NCS is located at the periphery, independent of the nucleolus. In some sections a few larger than average mitochondria were seen,

77

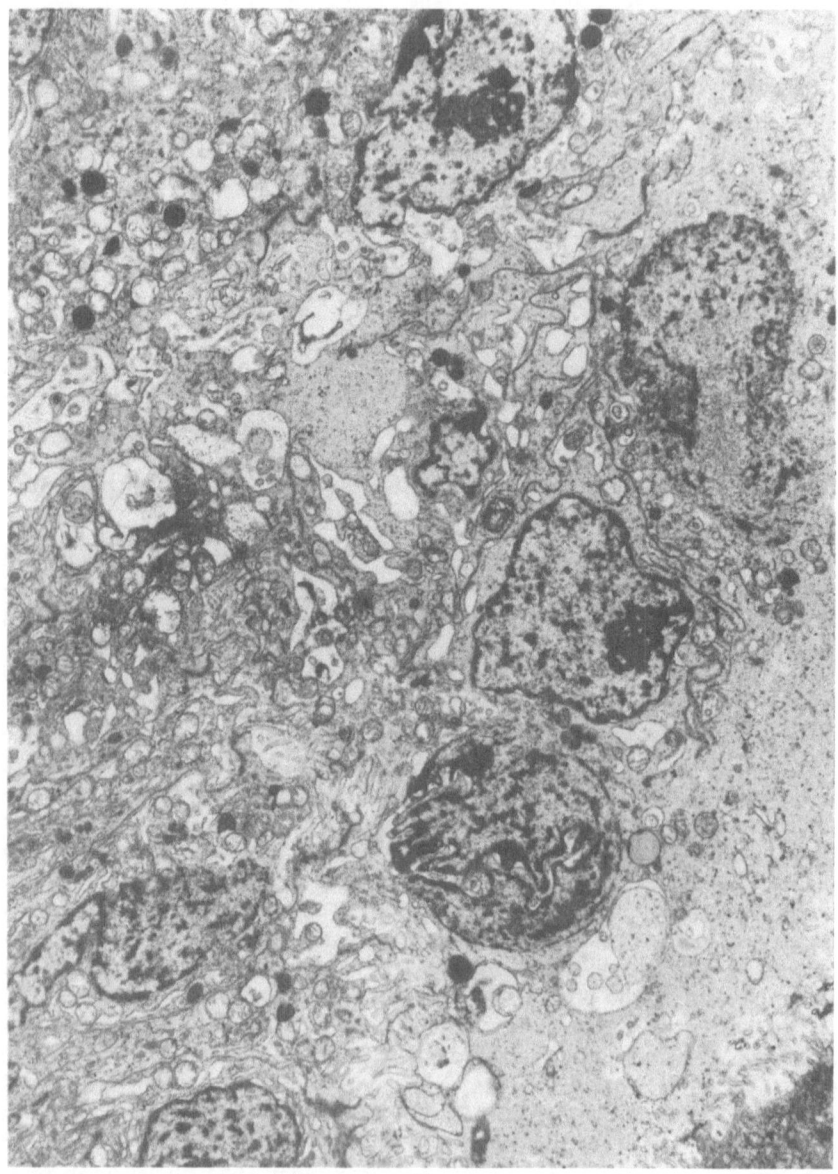

Figure 6.6 CLI-endometrium at day 12 showing degenerating cells (group ID/IID). Clumping of chromatin and swelling of all organelles and defects of the nuclear envelope and the cellular membranes are characteristic signs (× 8500)

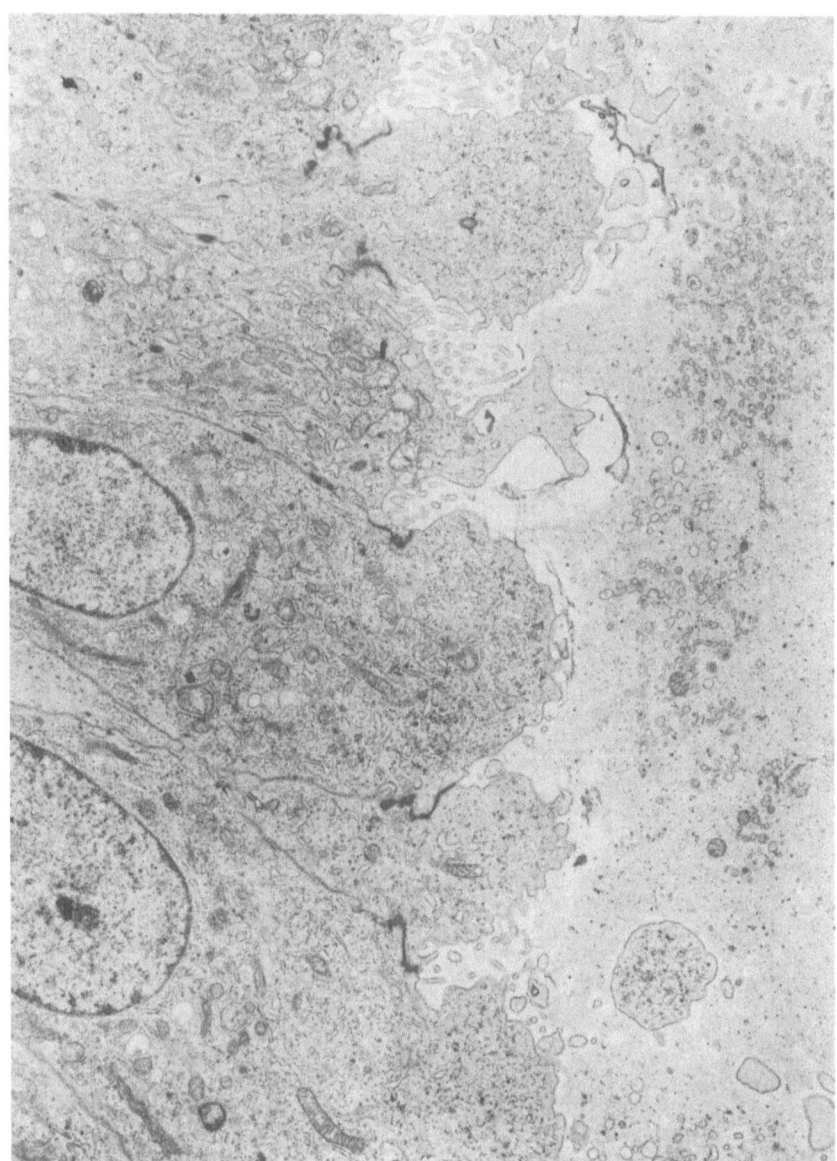

Figure 6.7 Still proliferating epithelium at day 8 after ovulation in a CLI cycle. The picture resembles the late proliferative to early secretory phase of a normal menstrual cycle (= group IA) (×7820)

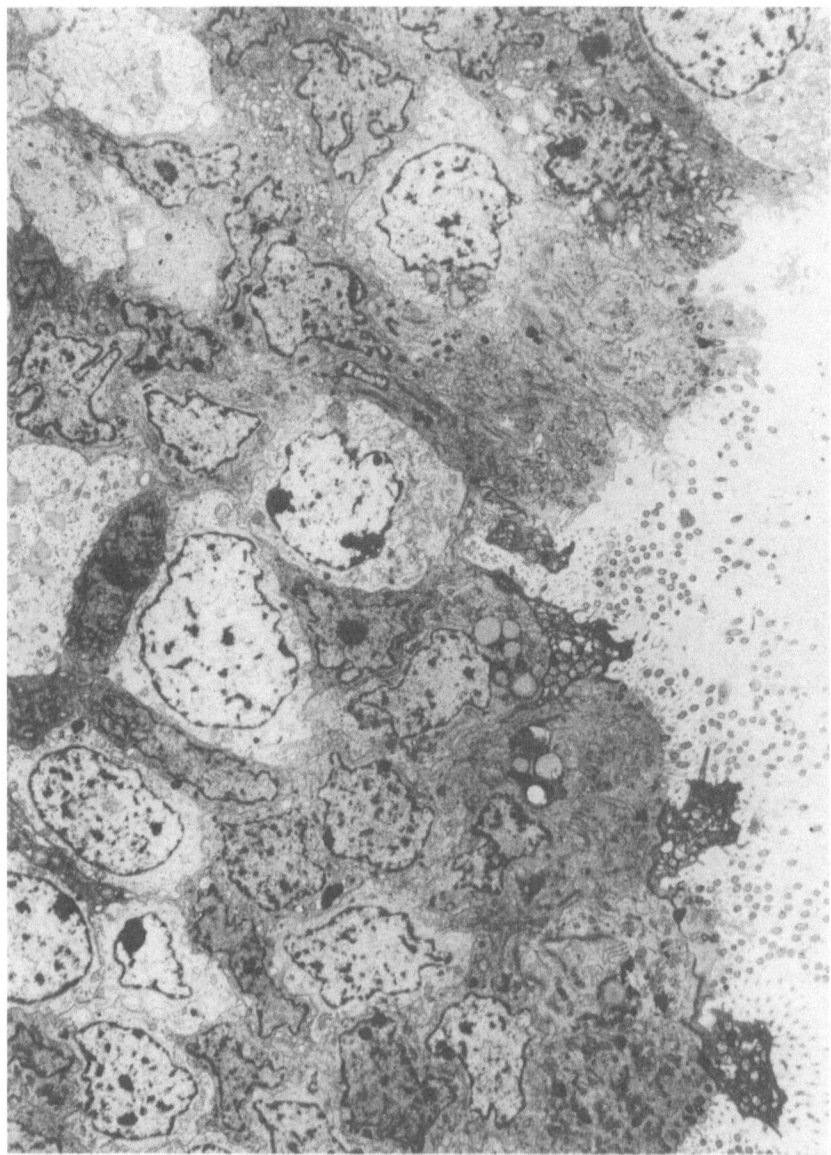

Figure 6.8 Mixed differentiation of group II glandular epithelium at day 8 after ovulation in a CLI cycle. Many ciliated cells and electron-light cells (= group IIB) are mixed with typical epithelial cells showing well-developed organelles and partly annulate lamellae (= group IIA). Only one electron-dense cell is seen on the left border (group IIC) (× 2375)

but typical giant mitochondria were absent. The Golgi complexes are moderately grown, forming small vesicles. The glycogen content is subnormal, and confluent patches are found very rarely in the apical or basal cytoplasm.

In addition to these so-called 'typical' epithelial cells the glandular epithelium contains electron-light cells (group IIB), of which the portion of ciliated cells has increased up to 50%. The ultrastructural features of the 'Helle Zellen' are characterized by an electron-lucent cytoplasm containing only few organelles such as dilated mitochondria, small Golgi complexes, and some rests of rER and free ribosomes. In general the nuclei are light with poorly developed chromatic material, but sometimes the nuclei are more electron-dense because of heterochromatic areas. These cells contain a larger number of well-differentiated mitochondria with an average of five to eight cristae intermitochondriales, while the other cytoplasmic organelles are poorly developed with signs of swelling and disorganization.

In contrast to this type of electron-light cells, other areas of the glandular epithelium are composed of dark, electron-dense cells (group IIC). The karyoplasm is heterochromatic, and the cytoplasm contains many free ribosomes, widened smooth and rough ER, secretory vesicles, and many small mitochondria with well-differentiated substructures. Dispersed spots of glycogen are present.

In addition – in all specimens of all patients – another type of cell showing various signs of degeneration is found (group ID/IID). The basal lamina is irregularly convoluted, the intercellular membranes have widened distance and the apical membranes are interrupted in many places. Almost 25% of the volume of the cells is pushed towards the lumen. The nuclei are irregularly shaped, and the nuclear membrane is often ruptured at its apical pole. ER, mitochondria and Golgi complexes are swollen and partly degenerated (Figure 6.9).

In contrast to the usual increasing differentiation of the stroma cells in the secretory phase of the menstrual cycle, the biopsies contain in general a poorly developed stroma. Although in areas with prismatic epithelium and beginning secretory activity some stroma cells with beginning predecidual transformation are found, spindle-shaped cells dominate, embedded in a dense network of fibrils (Figure 6.10). The cells are elongated, containing a heterochromatic nucleus with clumping of chromatin especially near the nuclear envelope. The cytoplasm is sparse, showing a compact Golgi complex, and few small mitochondria and few membranes of the smooth and rough ER.

The cells with beginning predecidual transformation contain an euchromatic, round shaped nucleus with one or two nucleoli. The nuclear–cytoplasmic ratio has increased in favour of the cytoplasm. Golgi complexes are moderately developed, and the membranes of the smooth and rough ER are widened. Characteristic endometrial "Körnchenzellen" – containing relaxin – cannot be observed. The ground substance is homogeneously stained, surrounding many filamentary elements.

To demonstrate the different cell types of the uterine mucosa of day 8 after ovulation of CLI patients a schematic overview is given in Figure 6.5.

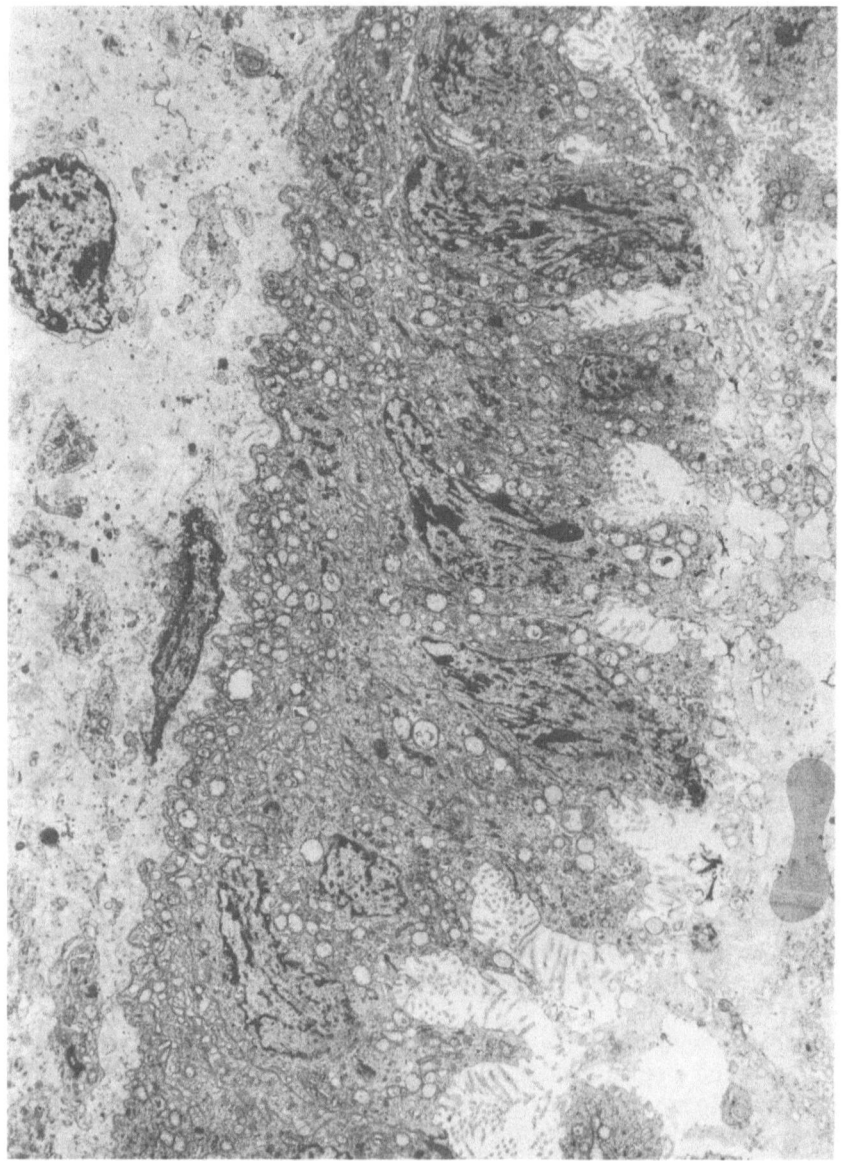

Figure 6.9 Endometrium of a CLI cycle at day + 8 after ovulation showing different degrees of degeneration. Clumping of chromatin in the nuclei, swelling of mitochondria and Golgi complexes as well as shrinking of the cells with widened intercellular distances are uniformly seen (× 5830)

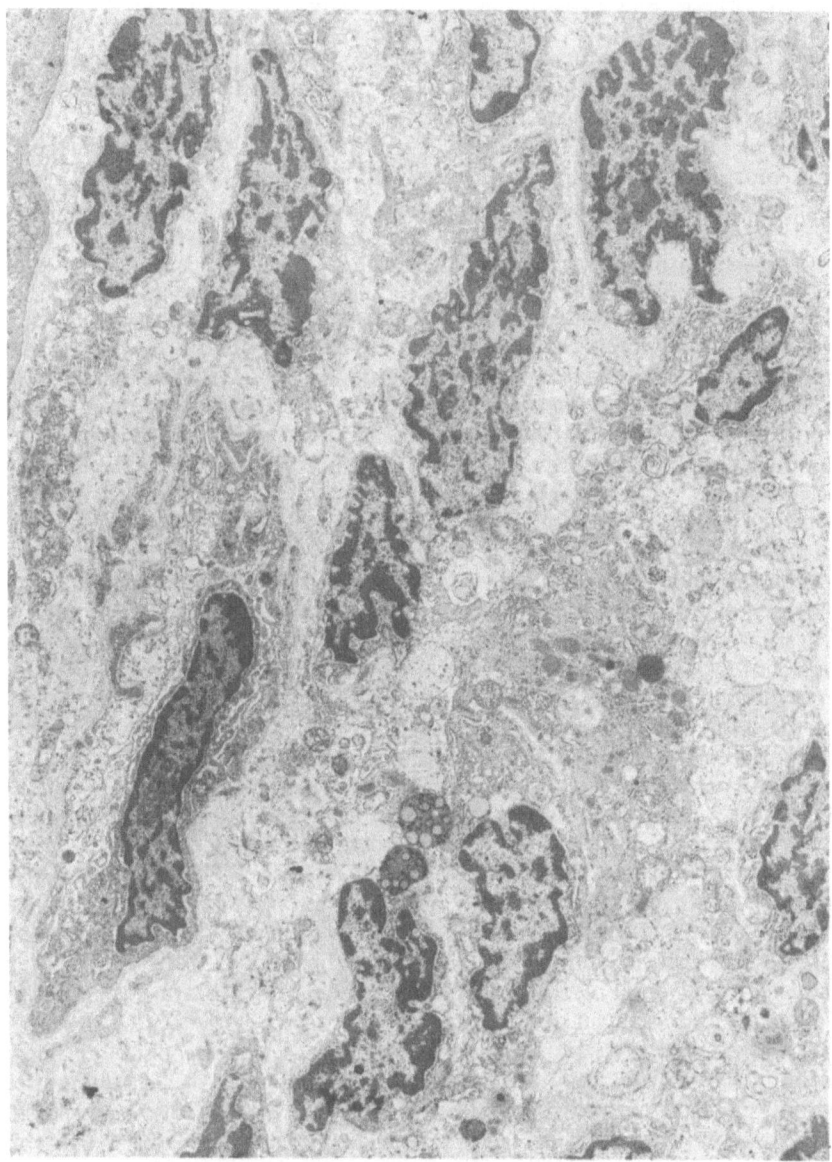

Figure 6.10 Undifferentiated stroma of endometrium at day 8 after ovulation of a CLI cycle. The stroma cells show irregularly shaped, heterochromatic nuclei and reduced cytoplasm, which contains very few organelles (×8655)

DISCUSSION

The interpretation of these ultrastructural findings must consider the functional morphological changes of the epithelium and the stroma. The following hypotheses may explain the described data:

(1) The delayed and insufficient morphological modulation during a cycle with CLI is caused by a more or less insufficient estrogen and/or progesterone secretion in the biopsy cycle.
(2) The differences of the ultrastructural features and the inhomogeneous morphology of the glandular epithelial cells are the result of an inadequate hormonal stimulation, which lasted for more than one cycle.
(3) A combination of the pathomechanism (1) and (2) can explain the whole spectrum of the morphological findings.

The specimens of group I are characterized by a mostly homogeneous morphology. The differences to the normal appearance of day 12 endometrium are primarily the reduced volume of cytoplasm and, in addition, reduced apical protrusions, and narrowed lumina. The increase of the volume of the epithelial cells, the enlargement of apical protrusions and microvilli are supposed to be characteristic morphological signs of adequate estrogen stimulation[1-4]. Their lagging development is an indication for insufficient estrogen stimulation caused by reduced plasma levels or reduced sensibility of the cells.

The specimens of group II demonstrate a mixture of different cell types. The degree of morphological alterations varies in different biopsies and in different areas of the same biopsy. Some glands are predominantly composed of CLI-typical cells (group IIA), while others show mostly regressed epithelium (IIB,C,D). Typical for group IIA cells is the unusual S-folding[5] of the intercellular membranes even in the apical part of the cells. These formations may result from secretion of cytoplasmic material[3] leading to a reduced volume of the cells with shrinking of the intercellular membranes. The mostly heterochromatic karyoplasm may be an expression of minor transcription activity. Rough ER and mitochondria are increased in relation to the volume of the cells. Similar changes have been described after prolonged estrogen effect[6]. The proliferation of some parallel membranes of the rER indicates a transformation into annulate lamellae[7, 8]. Although this structure is present sometimes in an undisturbed cycle[9], in general it is induced by a combined estrogen–progestogen effect with progesterone deficiency and estrogen dominance[7, 10].

Another characteristic finding is an increase of electron-light cells (group IIB). Partly, they belong to ciliated cells with well-differentiated cytoplasm. But many of them show blown-up ER and Golgi-tubules, the nuclear membranes are ruptured in some areas, and the karyoplasm contains poor chromatic material. The mitochondria remain unaffected, even if the other organelles show striking regressive changes. This can be interpreted as an attempt of the cell to save the energy system as long as possible. The loss of polysomes and free ribosomes is responsible for the electron-light appearance of the cells. This is correlated with a reduced content of RNA, as already described[11]. 'Helle Zellen' are also believed to be dividing cells[12], which means that the ability to perform mitosis leads to a degenerating cell after failed segmentation[13, 14]. According to the literature electron-light cells are a sign of prolonged estrogen stimulation[6] as found for example in glandular cystic hyperplasia.

Another type of degeneration is seen in electron-dense cells with a hetero-chromatic nucleus, and a ribosome-rich cytoplasm, containing healthy or dilated organelles (group IIC). These cells were described under quingestanol influence[15], and classified as residual cells, which were not desquamated in the preceding menstruation. The cause could be disturbed lysosomal activity, which depends on a sufficient estrogen and progesterone level.

The autolytic cells (groups ID and IID) are an expression of exhaustion and involution, caused by reduced hormonal levels[16–18].

New TEM and SEM observations indicate that secretory substances, and especially lysosomes, which reach their maximum in the late proliferative phase, play an important role in sperm capacitation[19–21]. The reduction of these secretory products in the glandular lumen of a CLI cycle may be a factor which could interfere with fertility.

Additional factors – probably more important – are ultrastructural changes of the defect secretory phase. The endometrium of group I shows on day 22 continuing proliferation. The characteristic postovulatory trias of glycogen patches, giant mitochondria and NCS, is missing. The elongated nuclei and the euchromatic karyoplasm express continuing transcription as much as the large amount of polysomes and well-developed rER. As a result of continuing proliferation the secretory activity is insufficient. There is not enough glycogen available for the synthesis of mucin, mucopolysaccharides and glycopolysaccharides, and the large amount of ribosomes indicates an insufficient consumption of these structures[3, 22]. The nutrition of the blasto-cyst from day 18 to day 20 depends on secretory products of the uterine mucosa. Therefore it is likely that the changed quality and quantity of the secretory material in a CLI cycle cause infertility.

The NCS, which was seen in some cells characterized as CLI-typical (group IIA), develops only in estrogen-primed endometrium[8, 23–25] and depends on a sufficient progesterone stimulation[25, 26]. Estrogen deficiency interferes with normal development of the NCS, even with adequate progesterone levels[8]. This leads to the following hypotheses:

In group I the NCS is not developed as a result of absolutely or relatively low progesterone levels and/or as a result of insufficient estrogen priming in the proliferative phase.

In group II some nuclear channel systems are found in CLI-typical cells, but there is no correlation to giant mitochondria and glycogen patches. Prolonged estrogen influence may lead to prolonged use of intracellular glucose for ATP production. After a complete cell proliferation the glucose metabolism is changed to produce glycogen. This causes enlargement of the mitochondria, in which the hexokinase reaction takes place[3]. In addition, the well-developed smooth ER, which plays a role in synthesis and transport, may be also responsible for the lack of glycogen[27]. The stimulus to change the metabolic pathways is probably NCS-dependent. Inadequate progesterone levels may cause an insufficient or delayed development of NCS, resulting in a delayed formation of giant mitochondria and insufficient stimulation of other progesterone-related metabolic processes.

These functional and morphological changes could interfere with the implantation process. It was shown[29] that the blastocyst takes its energy from glycolysis while invading the epithelium. The distribution of glycogen in the mucosa reflects its functional importance. The epithelial cells of the superficial glands contain glycogen earlier and for a longer period (until day 26) in a normal cycle[29]. In a CLI cycle the glycogen content is reduced, the glandular epithelium is inhomogeneously differentiated, and the ciliated cells are increased, which are normally reduced around day 20/21[29]. It is possible that the increase up to 50% could interfere with the first contact and adhesion of the blastocyst, which may be propelled by continuous beating of the ciliae to the lower uterine segment. The large number of ciliated cells is also a sensitive parameter for the endocrine situation, i.e. a sign of insufficient progesterone levels and/or predominance of estrogen.

The invasion of the blastocyst into the uterine mucosa involves phagocytosis or autolysis of the epithelium. This process is facilitated by proteolytic enzymes of lysosomes[30], which are labilized by steroids[31], mainly progesterone[32]. This has been demonstrated in animal experiments[32, 33]. Therefore reduced labilization of lysosomal membranes and the decreased amount of lysosomes may be additional factors for functional disturbances in a CLI-endometrium. The lack of homogeneous decidual transformation of the stroma cells seems to be another important point. The electron-density of the ground substance indicates high viscosity and insufficient low molecular substances[34].

Bundles of fibres prove that a progesterone-specific inhibition of bundling has not occurred[35]. The differentiation of the stroma cells is rudimentary, and predecidual changes such as high cytoplasmic volume, well-developed Golgi complexes and smooth ER, which are important for incretory functions[35] are missing. Relaxin containing 'Körnchenzellen' could not be found in our material. Therefore the lack of relaxin causes reduced lysis of fibres and no hyperplasia of spiral arterioles at the implantation site[36, 37].

To explain the whole spectrum of morphological findings in CLI-endometrium, the mechanism of menstruation must be taken into consideration. It has been shown that the mucosa is only partly desquamated[38–40]. The residual surface epithelium connects with the growing cells of the zona basalis. This regeneration takes place until day 5 of the cycle and is apparently hormone-independent[39, 40]. The ability of regeneration has been proven ultrastructurally, because hyperhydration, swelling of mitochondria and Golgi complexes has been observed to be reversible[41].

The possible pathogenesis of the morphological changes in CLI-endometrium is demonstrated in Figure 6.11. After a normal menstrual cycle the first insufficient cycle causes insufficient proliferation. During inadequate luteal phase an estrogen predominance, due to insufficient progesterone levels, may lead to a continuous proliferative stimulus. This prevents the development of NCS and the differentiation of stroma cells. Missing relaxin

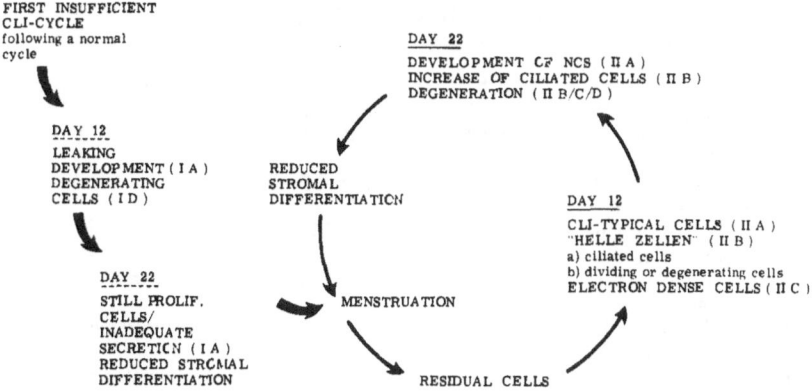

Figure 6.11 Pathogenesis of the morphological changes in CLI cycles

containing 'Körnchenzellen' lead to an inadequate desquamation. A lot of residual cells regenerate and are responsible for the inhomogeneous morphology of the following cycle (group II). A repeated estrogen dominance causes an increase of electron-light cells (IIB). Further studies with endocrine profiles of consecutive cycles are necessary to prove this hypothesis, that the degree of ultrastructural alterations of the endometrium correlates with the duration of hormonal disturbances and the number of endocrine-insufficient cycles.

References

1. Nilsson, O. (1958). Ultrastructure of mouse uterine surface epithelium under different oestrogen influence. Early effect of oestrogen administered to spayed animals. *J. Ultrastruct. Res.*, **2**, 185b
2. Nilsson, O. (1958). Late effect of oestrogen administered to spayed animals. *J. Ultrastruct. Res.*, **2**, 199b
3. Themann, H. and Schünke, W. (1963). Die Feinstruktur der Drüsenepithelien des menschlichen Endometriums. In: Schmidt-Mathiessen, H. *Das normale menschliche Endometrium.* (Stuttgart: Georg Thieme Verlag)
4. Wetzstein, R. and Wagner, H. (1960). Elektronenmikroskopische Untersuchungen am menschlichen Endometrium. *Anat. Anz.*, **108**, 362
5. Hofmeister, H. and Schulz, H. (1961). Lichtoptische und elektronenoptische Befunde am Endometrium der geschlechtsreifen Frau während der Proliferations- und der Sekretionsphase unter besonderer Berücksichtigung der Faserstrukturen. *Beitr. Pathol. Anat.*, **124**, 415
6. Wessel, W. (1961). Die glandulär-cystische Hyperplasie des menschlichen Endometriums im elektronenmikroskopischen Bild. *Virchows Arch. Pathol.*, **334**, 181
7. Ancla, M. and de Brux, J. (1965). Occurrence of intranuclear tubular structures in the human endometrium during the secretory phase and of annulate lamellae in hyperestrogenic states. *Obstet. Gynecol.*, **26**, 1
8. Ancla, M., de Brux, J., Belaisch, J. and Musset, R. (1964). Influence de l'équilibre oestrogène-progestérone sur les ultrastructures de l'endomètre humain. I. Morphologie et évolution de corpuscules intranucléaires presents dans les cellules glandulaires de l'endomètre sous l'effet de la norethistérone et dans les stérilités essentielles. *Gynecol. Obstet.*, **63**, 239

9. Ancla, M., de Brux, J., Musset, R. and Bret, J. A. (1967). Étude au microscope électronique de l'endomètre humain dans differentes conditions d'équilibre hormonal. *Acta. Anat. Pathol. Hors Serie*, **15**, 136

10. Ancla, M., de Brux, J., Belaisch, J. and Musset, R. (1964). Influence de l'équilibre oestrogène-progésterone sur les ultrastructures de l'endomètre humain. II. Lamelles annelées intracytoplasmiques dans le cellules glandulaires au cours des états hyperestrogèniques. *Gynecol. Obstet.*, **63**, 365

11. Jakubovits, A. (1955). Experimentelle Beiträge zum Problem der sog. Hellen Zellen der Gebärmutterschleimhaut. *Z. Geburtsh. Gynäkol.*, **142**, 313

12. Fuchs, M. (1959). Über die "hellen Zellen" im Epithel der menschlichen Uterusschleimhaut. *Acta Anat.*, **39**, 244

13. Rotter, W. and Eigner, J. (1949/50). Über Degenerationsformen der hellen Zellen (Feyrter) des Endometriums. *Frankf. Z. Pathol.*, **61**, 92

14. Sarbach, W. (1955). Über helle Zellen im Endometrium unter besonderer Berücksichtigung der glandulär-cystischen Hyperplasie. *Gynaecologia*, **139**, 356

15. Flowers, C. E., Wilborn, W. H. and Enger, J. (1974). Effects of quingestanol acetate on the histology, histochemistry and ultrastructure of the human endometrium. *Am. J. Obstet. Gynecol.*, **120**, 589

16. Ratzenhofer, M. and Schmid, K. O. (1953). Über die Involutionsvorgänge am Drüsenepithel bei in Blüte befindlicher glandulär-cystischer Hyperplasie. *Ref. Zbl. allg. Path. und path. Anat.*, **90**, 150

17. Schmid, K. O. (1968). Über ungewöhnliche Epithelveränderungen und Rückbildungsvorgänge der Corpusmucosa infolge abnormer Hormonzufuhr. *Arch. Gynäkol.*, **205**, 466

18. Schmid, K. O. and Dapunt, O. (1968). Atypische Organwirkungen sogenannter Ovulationshemmer nach bilateraler Nephrektomie sowie ungewöhnliche Endometriumveränderungen während azyklischer Dauertherapie wegen chronischer Myelose. *Z. Geburtsh. Gynäkol.*, **168**, 268

19. Barberini, F., Sartori, S., Motta, P. and van Blerkom, J. (1978). Changes in the surface morphology of the rabbit endometrium related to the estrous and progestational stages of the reproductive cycle. *Cell Tissue Res.*, **190**, 207

20. Hafez, E. S. E. (1977). Kinetics of luminal secretions in the female reproductive tract. Ultrastructural and physiological parameters. *Acta Anat.*, **97**, 143

21. Motta, P. M. and van Blerkom, J. (1975). A scanning electron microscopic study of rabbit spermatozoa in the female reproductive tract following coitus. *Cell Tiss. Res.*, **163**, 29

22. Wessel, W. (1960). Das elektronenmikroskopische Bild menschlicher endometrialer Drüsenzellen während des Zyklus. *Z. Zellforsch.*, **51**, 633

23. Kohorn, E. I., Rice, S. I. and Gordon, M. (1970). *In vitro* production of nucleolar channel system by progesterone in human endometrium. *Nature*, **228**, 671

24. Luginbuhl, W. H. (1968). Electron microscopic study of the effects of tissue culture on human endometrium. *Am. J. Obstet. Gynecol.*, **103**, 192

25. Pryse-Davies, J., Ryder, T. A. and MacKenzie, M. L. (1979). *In vivo* production of the nucleolar channel system in post menopausal endometrium. *Cell Tiss. Res.*, **203**, 493

26. Feldhaus, F. J., Themann, H., Wagner, H. and Verhagen, A. (1977). Feinstrukturelle Untersuchungen über das Nuclear-Channel-System im menschlichen Endometrium. *Arch. Gynäkol.*, **223**, 195

27. Coimbra, A. and Leblond, C. P. (1966). Sites of glycogen synthesis of rat liver cells as shown by electron microscope radioautography after administration of glucose-H^3 *J. Cell. Biol.*, **30**, 151

28. Dallenbach-Hellweg, G. (1963). Endometrium und Nidation. In Schmidt-Mathiessen, H. (ed.) *Das normale menschliche Endometrium*. (Stuttgart: Georg Thieme Verlag)

29. Ferenczy, A. (1977). Surface ultrastructural response of the human lining epithelium to hormonal environment. Scanning electron microscopic study. *Acta. Cytol. (Baltimore)*, **21**, 566

30. Parkening, T. A. (1976). An ultrastructural study of implantation in the golden hamster. II. Trophoblastic invasion and removal of the uterine epithelium. *J. Anat.*, **122**, 211

31. Abraham, R., Hendy, R., Dougherty, W. J., Fulfs, J. C. and Goldberg, L. (1970). Participation of lysosomes in early implantation in the rabbit. *Exp. Molec. Pathol.*, **13**, 329

32. Bareither, M. C. and Verhage, H. G. (1979). Progesterone induced secretory release in cat endometrium. *J. Cell. Biol.*, **376a,**
33. Kirchner, C. (1972). Uterine protease activities and lysis of the blastocyst covering in the rabbit. *J. Embryol. Exp. Morphol.*, **28,** 177
34. Dallenbach-Hellweg, G. (1969). *Histopathologie des Endometriums.* (New York, Berlin, Heidelberg: Springer Verlag)
35. Liebig, W. and Stegner, H. E. (1977). Die Dezidualisation der endometrialen Stromazelle. *Arch. Gynäkol.*, **223,** 19
36. Dallenbach-Hellweg, G. (1976). Morphologisch faßbare Grundlagen a) der normalen Menstruation und ihrer Störungen, b) der Nidation, c) der Placentaablösung unter der Geburt. *Verh. Deutsch. Ges. Pathol.*, **60,** 375
37. Themann, H. (1976). Wissenschaftliche Sitzung der Sektion Gynäkopathologie: Lyso-somenbedingte physiologische und pathologische Gewebsaufs lösung im Corpusen-dometrium und im Bereich der Plazenta: die Ultrastruktur der endometrialen Körnchen-zellen. *Verh. Dtsch. Ges. Pathol.*, **60,** 373
38. Bartelmez, G. W. and Baltimore, D. (1957). The phases of the menstrual cycle and their interpretation in terms of the pregnancy cycle. *Am. J. Obstet. Gynecol.*, **74,** 5
39. Ferenczy, A. (1977). Studies on the cytodynamics of experimental endometrial regeneration in the rabbit. *Am. J. Obstet. Gynecol.*, **128,** 536
40. Ferenczy, A. (1976). Studies on the cytodynamics of human endometrial regeneration. *Am. J. Obstet. Gynecol.*, **124,** 582
41. Sengel, A. and Stoebner, P. (1970). Ultrastructure de l'endomètre humain normal. II. Les glandes. *Z. Zellforsch.*, **109,** 26

Discussion

Braendle	If I understood you correctly, your conclusions were that your data reflect the deficiency of steroid action. Is there any additional information which we could not have obtained by measuring steroid levels?
Schweppe	One patient who had a luteinized unruptured follicle syndrome, as confirmed ultrasonographically, was followed in the next cycle, and then she ovulated as confirmed by laparoscopy with sufficient progesterone levels in the luteal phase. The endometrial biopsy, however, showed exactly the same mixed pattern as in the cycle before, despite the normal progesterone secretion. I think that local circumstances must be taken into consideration, and it takes probably more than one or two endocrine-sufficient cycles to obtain a healthy-looking, normal-developing endometrium.
Insler	I would like to add some basic information. We tried to culture endometrial cells in a long-term culture, which showed the presence of estrogen and progesterone receptors. The addition of estrogen or progesterone to the culture medium, however, did not affect the growth of the cells; neither did it change the morphological appearance. Therefore, the response to hormonal levels is present only when the cells are in tissue and not in culture.
Breckwoldt	Cells in culture will respond in different ways to different agents. If you keep endometrial cells in culture and add progesterone or testosterone, you are able to slow down protein synthesis. If you add estrogens, you keep the protein synthesis going, unless you use pharmacological amounts which will markedly decrease the protein synthesis of the cells.
Köhler	If you add first estrogen and then progesterone to endometrial cells, you can provoke the nuclear channel system, the specific transformation of the nucleus.

Section 2
Diagnosis

7
Luteal phase inadequacy: problems of diagnostic routine*

J. S. E. DERICKS-TAN, H. KUHL AND H.-D. TAUBERT

Luteal phase inadequacy should be suspected in patients with primary infertility or in those having suffered repeated miscarriages, who menstruate spontaneously and relatively regularly, even though the intermenstrual interval may be shortened or lengthened, respectively.

The mean age of patients with luteal phase inadequacy tends to be somewhat higher than that of women with anovulatory infertility. In a recent review (Haiges and Taubert, unpublished observation), only 28% of the patients with luteal phase inadequacy were found to be below the age of 30 years, as compared to 78% in anovulatory women.

There are no typical symptoms or complaints associated with luteal phase inadequacy, except for the fact that the afflicted women have difficulties in conceiving or are prone to miscarry during the first trimester of pregnancy.

Premenstrual spotting is not a constant symptom, as it has often been claimed, and it is not seldom of cervical rather than endometrial origin. As this type of bleeding can be caused by a cervical focus of endometriosis, it should alert the examiner to the possibility that there is pelvic endometriosis, too.

A haematological or metabolic disorder, and infectious disease, particularly tuberculosis, should be excluded by appropriate tests. Special care should be taken not to overlook a case of clinically unapparent hypothyroidism. A determination of tri-iodothyronine (T3), thyroxine (T4), and TSH should, therefore, be a part of the diagnostic routine, and this should eventually be supplemented by a TRH-stimulation test.

It cannot be emphasized enough that other possible causes of infertility should carefully be ruled out, even if the diagnosis of luteal phase inadequacy has been established beyond reasonable doubt. It has been our experience that in nearly every other patient out of a group of 168 women with luteal phase inadequacy, one or more than one additional cause of infertility could be demonstrated. In particular, women with luteal phase inadequacy seem

---

* This article was conceived as an addition to the papers presented at the workshop.

to be predisposed to have cervical dysmucorrhoea also (Steinmüller and Taubert, unpublished observation). It is, therefore, mandatory to perform a post-coital test, to obtain a spermiocytogram of the husband, and to test the patency of the Fallopian tubes by means of a hysterosalpingography or pelviscopy.

As the ultimate causes of luteal phase inadequacy remain unknown, there is as yet no specific test to establish the diagnosis. The production of prolactin by cultured predecidual endometrial cells obtained by biopsy has been claimed to be lower in insufficient as compared to normal cycles[1]. This principally attractive, albeit complicated method is, however, as yet not applicable to clinical practice.

BASAL BODY TEMPERATURE

Most of the presently used methods for the diagnosis of luteal phase inadequacy are based on a direct or indirect measurement of progesterone. Even in present clinical practice, the diagnosis of luteal phase inadequacy is often made just on the basis of a short or otherwise atypical hyperthermic phase, although it has been well documented that the basal body temperature (BBT) does not reflect the quality of luteal function, as expressed by serum progesterone, very accurately. Luteal phase inadequacy should, however, be suspected when the hyperthermic shift is of less than 10 days duration (Figure 7.1), shows a slow 'staircase'-like pattern of increase, or the rise of the BBT is so indistinct as to raise the question whether ovulation has occurred or not.

A clearly recognizable shift in the BBT is usually seen when serum progesterone exceeds the level of 3 ng/ml serum[2], but it fails to occur in some

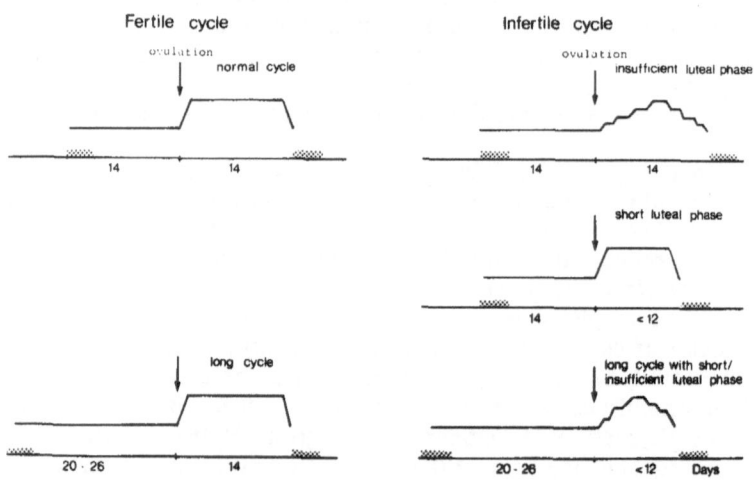

Figure 7.1 Schematic diagram of various types of biphasic basal body temperature (BBT) curves in cycles from fertile (left panel) and infertile women with luteal phase inadequacy (right panel)

women although the secretion of progesterone by the corpus luteum appears normal, at least as reflected by its concentration in peripheral blood[3, 4]. The reason for this discrepancy is not known. There is, however, some evidence that the metabolization of progesterone may be involved in the thermo-genetic effect, as it was shown that with regard to the elevation of BBT, one of the metabolites of progesterone, pregnane-3α-ol-20-one, is more effective and has a shorter time of latency as compared to progesterone[5, 6]. It is conceivable that this metabolic step may be impaired by various factors, e.g. by corticosteroids which are known to depress BBT[7]. Moreover, the thermo-genetic effect of progesterone is dependent on the previous exposure to a sufficient amount of estrogen[8].

Even though the measurement of the BBT must be considered to be a rather unreliable tool, a hyperthermic phase of less than 11 days duration has to be considered as fairly good evidence of luteal phase inadequacy[9].

ENDOMETRIAL BIOPSY

A well-timed endometrial biopsy performed 1–2 days (i.e. day 26 or 27 of a 28-day cycle) prior to the onset of menstruation can demonstrate endometrial secretory inadequacy. The rationale for choosing the premenstrual period rather than the period of nidation does not need to be reiterated as it has been amply discussed by Dr Dallenbach in the preceding Section (page 61). The BBT should be recorded during the cycle of investigation, as it is nearly indispensable for proper timing of the biopsy, particularly if there is a noticeable variation with respect to the day of ovulation in subsequent cycles. The date of the preceding, and especially of the subsequent, menstruation, the presumptive day of ovulation, and the characteristics of the BBT record should be documented, and this information should be made available to the histologist examining the specimen. The dating of the endometrium according to the criteria of Noyes et al.[10] can be facilitated by demonstrating the pre-ovulatory LH peak by serial measurement in serum or morning-urine specimen (Figure 7.2). The diagnosis of luteal phase inadequacy should not be considered to be definite unless the finding of endometrial inadequacy has been confirmed by another biopsy taken within 2–3 cycles.

It is of paramount importance that the endometrial specimen is obtained from the fundal portion of the uterine cavity, and it should represent the full thickness of the mucosal layer. Tissue specimen taken from lower portions of the uterine cavity can mislead the examiner into a false diagnosis of endometrial secretory inadequacy, since endometrium taken from that location does not show the same full-blown pattern of secretory transformation as samples obtained from the fundus.

Although the endometrial biopsy is an invasive diagnostic method, the discomfort experienced by the patient is minimal if some precautions are observed. A local anaesthetic, e.g. 2% solution of xylocaine, can be sprayed upon the cervix prior to applying the tenaculum; and the traction on the uterus, and the insertion of a Novak or Miles curette, should be performed

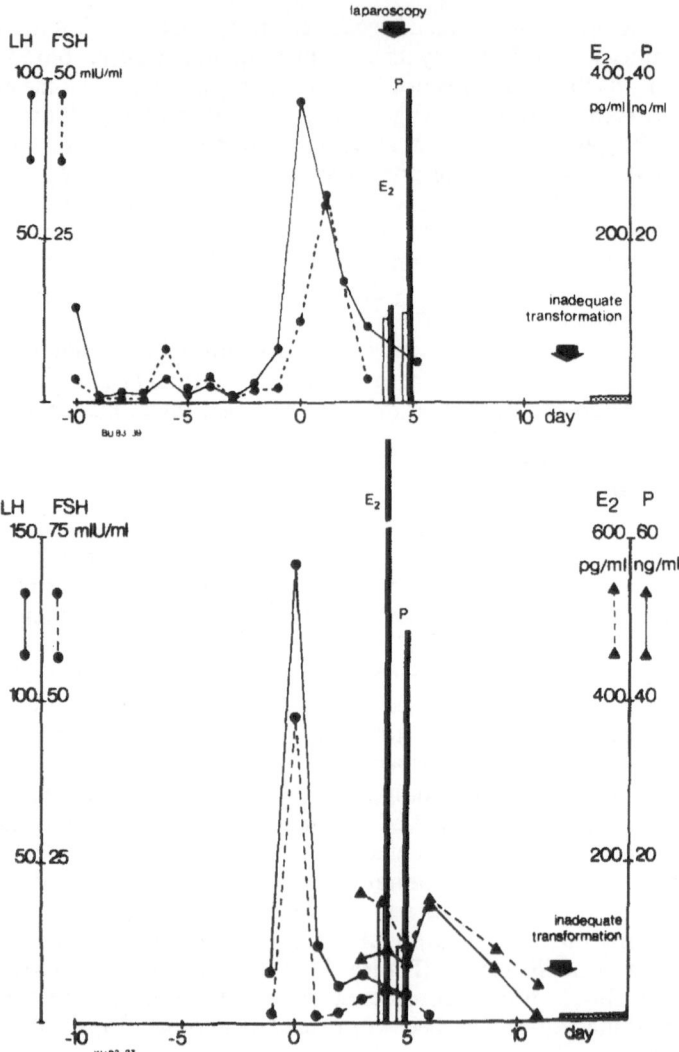

Figure 7.2 Dating of endometrial biopsy by serial determination of LH (solid line) and FSH (dotted line) in early morning urine in two patients with an inadequate luteal phase. The concentration estradiol (E2: ▲----▲) and progesterone (P: ▲——▲) in serum and in peritoneal fluid (open bars = serum; solid bars = peritoneal fluid) at the time of laparoscopy 4 days after the LH peak in urine, is also depicted. In the upper frame the FSH peak does not coincide with the LH peak

gently. In order to avoid episodes of hypotension or syncope due to vagal hyperstimulation, 0.25–0.5 mg atropine sulphate is administered i.v. or i.m. prior to the procedure. If the patient had unprotected intercourse in midcycle, an early pregnancy should be ruled out by measuring hCG in serum on the day of biopsy or the day before, even though it seems to be exceptional to disturb a pregnancy by the trauma of biopsy[11].

In a series of 143 consecutive biopsies performed by one of the authors only two patients complained about severe pain during the procedure. Although this incidence is low, it should be emphasized that cervical stenosis or hyper-flexion of the uterus will prevent the insertion of the Novak curette in some patients unless the cervical canal is dilated to some degree under general anaesthesia.

A normal secretory transformation of the endometrium was found in only 24% of 143 infertile women[12] showing an atypical BBT during the biopsy cycle, as compared to 53% presenting an inconspicuous hyperthermic phase. In the remaining patients of each group, the endometrium was out of phase or proliferative. This shows clearly that endometrial secretory inadequacy may be found in nearly every other infertile woman with an apparently normal, biphasic BBT record. On the other hand, there is roughly a 3 out of 4 chance that the impression gained by the interpretation of an atypical temperature record will be confirmed by the result of the biopsy. It could hence be argued with some justification that a biopsy should not be manda-tory if the BBT is grossly abnormal. It should also, however, be performed in such a case, when a patient fails to conceive after several cycles of therapy, in order to determine whether the mode of treatment succeeded in correcting the endometrial defect, as it has unequivocally been shown that the endo-metrial biopsy – with certain exceptions[13] – reflects the functional state of both the ovarian and the endometrial cycle, and can be used to determine adequacy of therapy.

A comparison of at least three BBT records obtained within a 6-month period around the cycle of biopsy revealed that the finding of an atypical temperature record tended to be more consistent than apparently normal hyperthermic phases. Consequently, some cases of luteal phase inadequacy may not be recognized if one relies too much on a normally appearing basal temperature record.

HORMONAL MEASUREMENTS

Steroid hormones

The finding of an out-of-phase endometrium is often caused by insufficient stimulation by progesterone and, possibly, estrogens. It could, therefore, be argued that the direct measurement of progesterone in serum should be substituted for the endometrial biopsy or at least used as an additional diagnostic parameter.

A single measurement of progesterone obtained during the hyperthermic phase can be helpful in determining whether a particular cycle is ovulatory or not if the serum level[2] exceeds 3 ng/ml. Since the serum level of progester-one is subject to considerable day-to-day and short-term fluctuations, single or double determinations performed during the height of the luteal phase and at the time of biopsy are without value for the diagnosis of luteal phase inadequacy[14, 15]. Whenever progesterone is used as a diagnostic parameter for assessing luteal adequacy, at least three blood specimens should be obtained during the mid-luteal phase, i.e. 9 to 5 days prior to the onset of the next menses. Each of the blood samples should contain more than 10 ng/ml progesterone. The most practical way of measuring progesterone and estradiol in clinical routine is probably to take a blood specimen every other day beginning after the rise of the BBT (e.g. Monday, Wednesday, Friday, Monday, etc.). The evaluation of the results can be performed by one of the following methods:

The calculation of the area under the curve (AUC) provides an index of the sum of progesterone action during the luteal phase, and reduces the chance of misinterpretations due to periodic fluctuations of progesterone secretion. The method has, however, a disadvantage in that it does not allow one to distinguish a short luteal phase from a luteal phase of ordinary duration with insufficient secretion of progesterone. Moreover, the calculation of the AUC requires exact dating of the time of ovulation in order to avoid an over- or underestimation of secretory capacity of the corpus luteum.

As an alternative, the calculation of a 'progesterone index' has also been proposed[16] to facilitate the interpretation of the results. As this method entails daily sampling of blood during the whole cycle, it is ill-suited to the needs of clinical practice.

It should, however, be noted that there is a lack of congruence between the laparoscopic demonstration of a corpus luteum, endometrial histology and serum progesterone in some instances[13]. This means that endometrial histology occasionally does not reflect cyclic ovarian function. This could be due to a defect of progesterone action on endometrial stroma[17] or reduced estradiol levels[18, 19], as it was reported that estradiol can induce progesterone receptors[20, 21]. Similarly, inadequate maturation of the endometrium seems to correlate with insufficient development of progestin receptor binding sites rather than with a decreased serum progesterone level[22], and a mid-luteal estradiol level of less than 150 pg/ml has been observed in patients with short luteal phase[19]. This means that the diagnostic value of progesterone measurements could probably be complemented by the assay of estradiol.

A certain relationship between plasma testosterone levels and the duration of the follicular and luteal phase has been demonstrated in women with ovulatory cycles[23], and prolonged follicular phase associated with a short luteal phase was found in patients with elevated plasma testosterone levels. Moreover, prednisone administration to ovulatory patients results in a shortening of the follicular phase and a lengthening of the luteal phase of the menstrual cycle[24]. This means that the estimation of testosterone levels in patients with luteal phase inadequacy could have therapeutic consequences.

Pituitary hormones

Reduced FSH secretion in the follicular phase[25-27], as well as a reduced FSH:LH ratio[27] in the presence of normal LH secretion may interfere with folliculogenesis and thus cause luteal phase inadequacy. Sporadic and recurrent luteal phase inadequacy have been shown to be characterized by an inappropriate ratio of FSH:LH during the whole cycle[28]. Similarly, imminent ovarian failure presenting with high FSH and LH levels can also bring about a defective luteal phase[29].

As this type of diagnostic investigation would require serial determination of FSH and LH, which are costly and time-consuming, no practical protocol for the study of aberrant gonadotropin secretion in luteal phase inadequacy has yet been proposed. Morning urine specimens which are easily obtained and stored frozen have been used to characterize the preovulatory LH peak as a point of reference for dating the endometrial biopsy. We have measured LH and FSH in morning-urine specimens obtained from infertile women following a standardized fluid-intake regime. This is exemplified by the data depicted in Figure 7.2. The 39-year-old woman (upper frame) underwent laparoscopy 4 days after the LH peak appeared in urine. A delayed FSH peak could be observed. No stigma could be demonstrated, but the progesterone level in the peritoneal fluid was 3 times that of serum. The histologic examination of the endometrial biopsy taken 12 days after the urinary LH peak and 1 day prior to the onset of menstruation revealed endometrial secretory inadequacy. As the estradiol concentration in the peritoneal fluid was not much higher than in serum, it was assumed that this patient suffered from luteal phase inadequacy associated with a cystic luteinized, unruptured follicle. For comparison, a normal serum to peritoneal fluid ratio for estradiol and progesterone ratio was found in a 27-year-old ovulatory woman with endometrial secretory inadequacy 4 days after an inconspicuous LH and FSH peak (Figure 7.2, lower frame).

It has been thoroughly discussed by Dr L'Hermite that hyperprolactinaemia may be a factor in the genesis of luteal phase inadequacy (page 49). The usefulness of PRL determinations has, however, been questioned, as a higher incidence of histologically inadequate endometrial biopsies had been found in normoprolactinaemic patients[30]. On the other hand, metoclopramide-induced hyperprolactinaemia has been shown to impair folliculogenesis and luteal function[31].

Whenever repeated measurements of PRL confirm, however, the diagnosis of overt or intermittent hyperprolactinaemia, and FSH and the FSH:LH ratio is low, luteal phase inadequacy is probably due to a dysfunction of the hypothalamo-pituitary axis. Intermittent or borderline hyperprolactinaemia is likely to be present when the i.v. injection of 10 mg metoclopramide is followed by a larger than 25-fold increase in serum PRL within 30 min.

Even though it is certainly not intended to make a claim for finality, we would like to propose the steps summarized in Figure 7.3 as a basis for a rational approach to the diagnosis of luteal phase inadequacy:

(1) The BBT record and a single determination of serum progesterone should suffice to distinguish ovulatory from anovulatory infertility.

(2) When luteal phase inadequacy is suspected as a cause of infertility, the BBT should be used as a guideline to obtain three to five blood specimens for the determination of progesterone, and for the timing of an endometrial biopsy.

(3) The differentiation of various possible causes of luteal phase inadequacy would require in addition serial measurements of PRL, LH, FSH, and

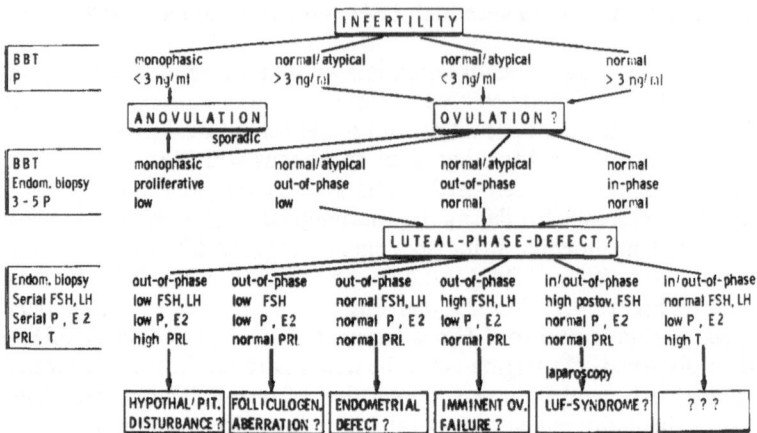

Figure 7.3 Diagrammatic presentation of diagnostic measures for the evaluation of luteal-phase inadequacy

estradiol during the luteal phase, and this can be complemented by ultrasound scannings as will be discussed by Dr Breckwoldt (page 103).

(4) Laparoscopy performed between day 17 and 19 of the cycle (10–12 days before the onset of the next menstruation) may be useful to exclude a LUF syndrome by demonstrating a stigma and a high ratio of progesterone and estradiol in peritoneal fluid to serum.

(5) Hypothyroidism and hyperandrogenaemia should be ruled out by appropriate tests in accordance with the circumstances in the individual case.

References

1. Daly, D. C., Maslar, I. A., Rosenberg, S. M., Tohan, N. and Riddick, D. H. (1981). Prolactin production by luteal phase defect endometrium. *Am. J. Obstet. Gynecol.*, **140**, 587

2. Israel, R., Mishell, D. R., Stone, S. C., Thorneycroft, I. H. and Moyer, D. L. (1972). Single luteal phase serum progesterone assay as an indicator of ovulation. *Am. J. Obstet. Gynecol.*, **112**, 1043

3. Johansson, E. D. B., Larsson-Cohn, U. and Gemzell, C. (1972). Monophasic basal body temperature in ovulatory menstrual cycles. *Am. J. Obstet. Gynecol.*, **113**, 933

4. Moghissi, K. S. (1976). Accuracy of basal body temperature for ovulation detection. *Fertil. Steril.*, **27**, 1415

5. Lauritzen, C. (1960). Gestagene, Gestagenmetaboliten und Basaltemperatur. *6. Symp. dtsch. Ges. Endokr.* **1959**, Springer Verlag Berlin-Göttingen-Heidelberg, p. 69

6. Lauritzen, C. (1961). Zur hormonellen Regelung der Körpertemperatur bei der Frau. *Geburtsch. Frauenheilk.*, **157**, 46

7. Lauritzen, C. (1957). Untersuchungen über den Einfluß von ACTH und Cortisonderivaten auf die basale Körpertemperatur der Frau. *Zbl. Gynäk.*, **79**, 1829

8. Schlösser, W. (1955). Beziehungen zwischen der Basaltemperatur und dem Funktionszustand des Endometriums nach exogener Hormonzufuhr. *Geburtsh. Frauenheilk.*, **15**, 917

9. Downs, K. A. and Gibson, M. (1983). Basal body temperature graph and the luteal phase defect. *Fertil. Steril.*, **40**, 466

10. Noyes, R. W., Hertig, A. T. and Rock, J. (1950). Dating the endometrial biopsy. *Fertil. Steril.*, **1**, 3
11. Cline, D. L. (1979). Unsuspected subclinical pregnancies in patients with luteal phase defect. *Am. J. Obstet. Gynecol.*, **134**, 438
12. Heil, B. and Taubert H.-D. (1984). Die Wertigkeit der Endometriumsbiopsie bei der Diagnose des Luteal-Phasen-Defekts (In preparation)
13. Perez, R. J., Plurad, A. V. and Palladino, V. S. (1981). The relationship of the corpus luteum and the endometrium in infertile patients. *Fertil. Steril.*, **35**, 423
14. Rosenberg, S. M. (1980). Inappropriateness of single mid-luteal progesterone for the diagnosis of corpus luteum defect (Letter). *Obstet. Gynecol.*, **56**, 267
15. Pachna, K. and Taubert, H.-D. (1980). Endometriumsbiopsie und Progesteronbestimmung in der Diagnostik von Zyklusstörungen. *Gynäkol. Prax.*, **4**, 433
16. Coutts, J. R. T., Adam, A. H. and Fleming, R. (1982). The deficient luteal phase may represent an anovulatory cycle. *Clin. Endocrinol.*, **17**, 389
17. Keller, D. W., Wiest, W. G., Askin, F. B., Johnson, L. W. and Strickler, R. C. (1979). Pseudocorpus luteum insufficiency: a local defect of progesterone action on endometrial stroma. *J. Clin. Endocrinol. Metab.*, **48**, 127
18. Driessen, F., Holwerda, P. J., Putte, S. C. J. v.d., Alsbach, G. P. J., Kroon, R. A. de and Kremer, J. (1980). Serum progesterone and estradiol concentrations in menstrual cycles with and without a delay in endometrial development. *Infertility*, **3**, 29
19. Goldstein, D., Zuckerman, H., Harpaz, S., Barkai, J., Geva, A., Gordon, S., Shalev, E. and Schwartz, M. (1982). Correlation between estradiol and progesterone in cycles with luteal phase deficiency. *Fertil. Steril.*, **37**, 348
20. Dodson, K. S., MacNaughton, N. C. and Coutts, J. R. T. (1975). Infertility in women with apparently ovulatory cycles. *Br. J. Obstet. Gynaecol.*, **82**, 615
21. Schmidt-Gollwitzer, M. (1978). Korrelation zwischen den Sexualsteroiden im Serum und im Endometrium, den östradiol- und progesteronbindenden Rezeptorproteinen und der Aktivität der 17ß-HSD während des mensuellen Zyklus. *Habilitationsschrift Berlin*
22. Laatikainen, T., Andersson, B., Kärkkäinen, J. and Wahlström, T. (1983). Progestin receptor levels in endometria with delayed or incomplete secretory changes. *Obstet. Gynecol.*, **62**, 592
23. Smith, K. D., Rodriguez-Rigau, L. J., Tcholakian, R. K. and Steinberger, E. (1979). The relation between plasma testosterone levels and the lengths of phases of the menstrual cycle. *Fertil. Steril.*, **32**, 403
24. Rodriguez-Rigau, L. J., Smith, K. D., Tcholakian, R. K. and Steinberger, E. (1979). Effect of prednisone on plasma testosterone levels and on duration of phases of the menstrual cycle in hyperandrogenic women. *Fertil. Steril.*, **32**, 408
25. Strott, C. A., Cargille, C. M., Ross, G. T. and Lipsett, M. B. (1970). The short luteal phase. *J. Clin. Endocrinol. Metab.*, **30**, 256
26. Sherman, B. M. and Korenman, S. G. (1974). Measurement of plasma LH, FSH, estradiol and progesterone in disorders of the human menstrual cycle: the short luteal phase. *J. Clin. Endocrinol. Metab.*, **38**, 89
27. Cook, C. L., Rao, Ch.V. and Yussman, M. A. (1983). Plasma gonadotropin and sex steroid hormone levels during early, midfollicular, and midluteal phases of women with luteal phase defects. *Fertil. Steril.*, **40**, 45
28. Aksel, S. (1980). Sporadic and recurrent luteal phase defects in cyclic women: comparison with normal cycles. *Fertil. Steril.*, **33**, 372
29. Rosenberg, S. M., Johnson, M. and Riddick, D. H. (1982). Luteal phase defect as a marker of imminent ovarian failure. *Obstet. Gynecol.*, **59**, 89S
30. Vanrell, J. A. and Balasch, J. (1983). Prolactin in the evaluation of luteal phase in infertility. *Fertil. Steril.*, **39**, 30
31. Kauppila, A., Leinonen, P., Vihko, R. and Ylöstalo, P. (1982). Metoclopramide-induced hyperprolactinemia impairs ovarian follicle maturation and corpus luteum function in women. *J. Clin. Endocrinol. Metab.*, **54**, 955

8
Endocrinological and sonographic data in normal and insufficient cycles

M. BRECKWOLDT AND F. GEISTHÖVEL

Before discussing endocrinological and sonographic findings in luteal insufficiency it seems appropriate to summarize briefly some relevant clinical and experimental data on the pathogenesis of the luteal dysfunction.

Normal luteal function is initiated after ovulation and completion of the luteinizing process of the granulosa and theca cells. Luteal function is terminated after a period of 12–16 days by continuous regression. This relatively short life span is only extended in conceptive cycles by recognition of hCG. Deficient progesterone secretion by the corpus luteum is associated with an inappropriate secretory transformation of the endometrium which may consequently impair or prevent nidation[1,2]. According to Sherman and Korenman[3,4] a short luteal phase is defined as a duration of 8 days or less from ovulation to menses. These authors also described a second type of luteal phase defect with normal duration yet reduced progesterone secretion. The second abnormality was termed the inadequate luteal phase. It has been suggested by many investigators that inappropriate patterns of circulating gonadotropins cause impairment of follicular development as reflected by decreased plasma estrogen levels during the proliferative phase. This abnormality may also lead to incomplete luteinization of the granulosa cells and consequently to an inadequate progesterone secretion[5,6]. Therefore, it has been emphasized that impairment of follicular development can result in inadequate luteal function. Sufficient FSH supply is essential for a normal luteal function. The critical role of FSH for proper development of granulosa cells has been demonstrated experimentally. Selective suppression of FSH with charcoal-extracted porcine follicular fluid (pFF) resulted in luteal dysfunction in rhesus monkeys[5,7]. After previous pFF treatment the luteal cells were almost unresponsive to hCG *in vitro*. This finding indicates the essential role of FSH for the synthesis of LH receptors.

From the clinical point of view luteal insufficiency is less well defined despite the fact that the diagnosis of corpus luteum insufficiency is frequently made in infertility patients. The incidence of luteal insufficiency in infertility patients varies between 3 and 30%. This wide range indicates the difficulties of proper evaluation and definition of luteal dysfunction. Clinical parameters used in diagnosing corpus luteum deficiency are medical history, BBT chart, progesterone determinations and eventually endometrial biopsies. These clinical parameters, however, are insufficient to discriminate between ovulatory cycles with inadequate luteal function and anovulatory cycles with luteinized unruptured follicles. Since ultrasonography has become a valuable tool in monitoring ovarian function this method has been applied to normal and insufficient ovarian cycles providing a better understanding of ovarian morphology, physiology and pathophysiology[8–11].

Figure 8.1 demonstrates a typical poly-follicular reaction of the right ovary at the initial phase of a normal cycle. These small multiple follicles can be visible from day 3 to day 13 after the onset of menses. Polymicro-follicular reaction as presented in Figure 8.1 is defined by the detection of at least three follicles of less than 10 mm in diameter per ovary, a leading or dominant follicle is undetectable, polymicro-follicular reaction is normally transitory with a duration of approximately 6 days.

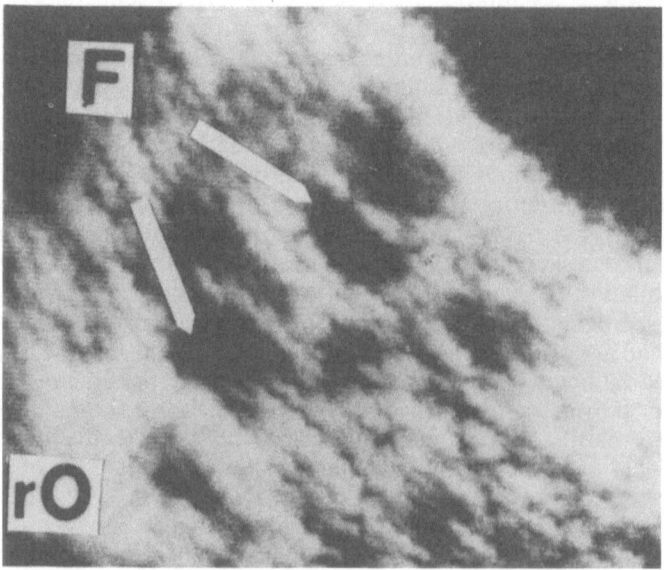

Figure 8.1 Polymicrofollicular reaction, multiple small follicles at the initial stage of a normal cycle

Persistent poly-follicular reaction, however, indicates a disturbed selection process since a dominant follicle is missing. Persistent poly-follicular reaction is a characteristic sonographic phenomenon in the polycystic ovary syndrome.

The selection of a dominant follicle is completed after one of the small follicles has grown to a cystic structure with a diameter of more than 10 mm. This follicle will develop and ovulate after reaching full maturity.

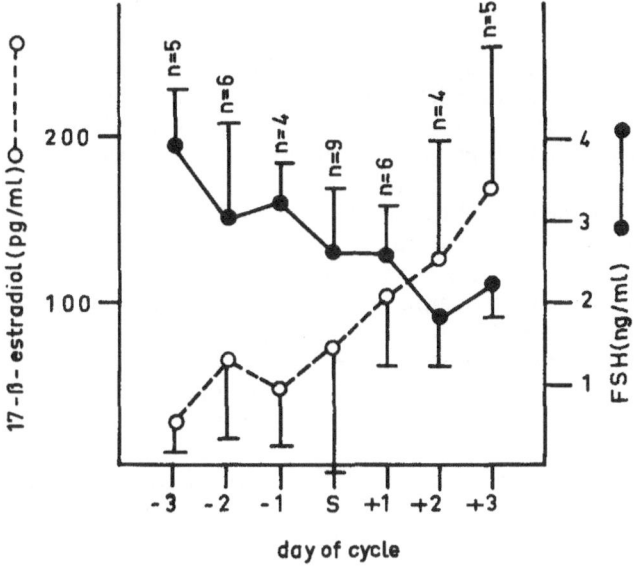

Figure 8.2 Mean plasma levels of FSH and estradiol-17β during the selective phase of the dominant follicle

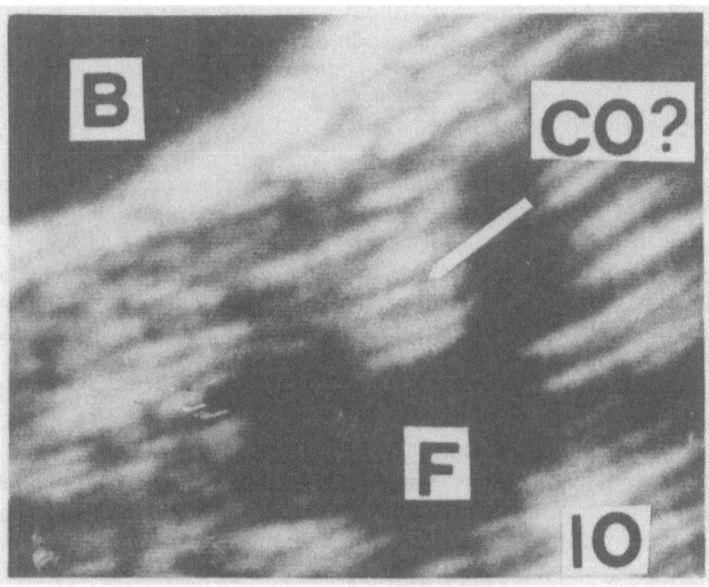

Figure 8.3 Sonographic presentation of a mature follicle with cumulus oophorus

Immediately after completion of the selection process serum estradiol levels start to rise progressively as the follicle matures. The FSH levels continue to decrease while the estrogen levels are rising, indicating that the leading follicle can be regarded as the main source of circulating estrogens. Mean plasma levels of FSH and estradiol-17β in correlation to the sonographic findings in apparently normal ovarian cycles are shown in Figure 8.2.

The sonographic findings of a preovulatory follicle with a maximal diameter of 22 mm are presented in Figure 8.3. The internal echoes seen at the top (CO) correspond to the cumulus oophorus.

Ovarian morphology immediately after ovulation on day 15 of a normal cycle is characterized by a rapid disappearance of the dominant follicle; no other solid or cystic structures are detectable. On day 18 a solid or cystic structure indicative of a corpus luteum appears in the ovary. Luteal structures may present in various forms, either as corpus luteum haemorrhagicum or as corpus luteum cysticum or as corpus luteum graviditatis with a diameter of 28.1 ± 6.7 mm. In conceptive cycles large corpus luteum cysts are detectable in most of the cases.

In 21 apparently normal cycles the length of the follicular phase was 14 ± 3.4 days. The selection phase took on average 9.1 ± 3.5 days. Diameters of the follicles being selected for ovulation were 10.3 ± 2.8 mm. Once selected it took normally 5–7 days for the follicle to become fully mature, reaching a diameter of 23.1 mm. The velocity of the daily growth was on average 2.5 mm and this seems to slow down as the maturation process proceeds, being 3 mm from day − 10 to − 3, reaching finally 1.5 mm from day − 1 to day 0. Day 0 indicates the day of the maximal follicular diameter.

The plasma progesterone levels in correlation to the follicular development during late follicular and early luteal phase are presented in Figure 8.4. Progesterone levels start to increase on day 0, reaching levels of 0.6 ng/ml increasing to 2.1 ng/ml on day 1, which indicates the day when the follicular structure has disappeared.

In normal ovarian cycles the length of the luteal phase was more or less constant, being 14.0 ± 1.0 days.

Figure 8.5 presents schematically various phases of normal ovarian function. Follicles with a diameter of less than 10 mm are regarded as immature; follicles with a diameter of 13–18 mm are defined as premature; follicles more than 18 mm diameter indicate follicular maturity. After disappearance of the leading follicle corpus luteum structures can be visible for a long period of time even after the function, namely the secretion of progesterone and estradiol, has ceased.

The morphological features of an inadequately developed follicle are poorly outlined cystic structures filled with irregular internal echoes, indicating a disturbed maturation.

In insufficient cycles folliculogenesis seems to be impaired as selection and maturation processes are disturbed. Sonographic observations present evidence that incompletely developed follicles with a diameter of 15 mm can rapidly regress, 6–8 days later a follicle of the same size may appear in the contralateral ovary and disappear without reaching full maturity. In most cases these poorly developed follicular cysts become atretic, the surrounding

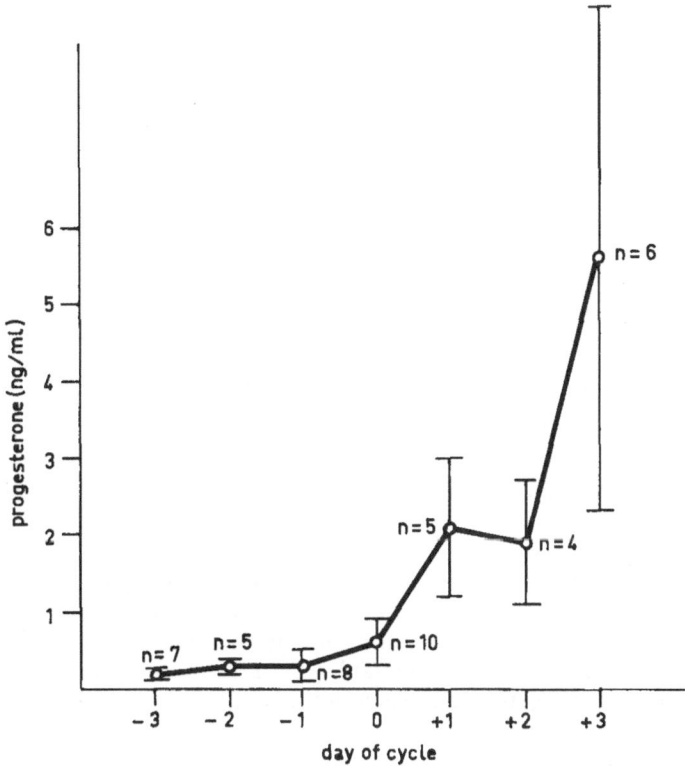

Figure 8.4 Mean progesterone levels ± SD during the periovulatory phase

granulosa cells may become more or less luteinized being capable of synthesizing and releasing progesterone to a small extent (Figure 8.6). Clinically this development can be misinterpreted as corpus luteum insufficiency.

In insufficient cycles the selection period is significantly longer than in physiological cycles, being 13.4±3.3 and 9.1±3.5 days respectively. In addition, the maximal follicular diameter is significantly smaller in insufficient cycles, being 16.9 mm versus 23.1 mm.

Figure 8.6 compares endocrinological data between physiological and insufficient cycles. Estradiol peaks in physiological cycles were observed mainly on day − 1 and also on day 0, which indicates the day of maximal follicular growth. In insufficient cycles, however, estradiol peaks were seen at various days of the periovulatory phase, reaching from day − 2 to day 5. Peak values of LH were detected on day − 1, day 0 and day 1 in physiological cycles. In the insufficient cycles, however, peak values of LH were seen from day − 3 to day 5 of the periovulatory phase. The distribution pattern of the progesterone increase discriminates clearly physiological from insufficient cycles.

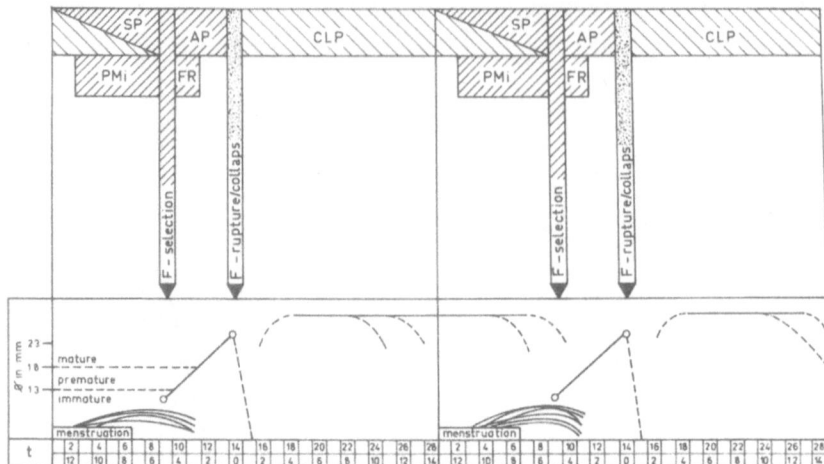

Figure 8.5 Schematic presentation of sonographic criteria characteristic for normal ovarian function

The data presented so far indicate that ultrasonography has become a useful additional instrument to monitor ovarian function. It is possible to detect the onset of follicular maturation and the selection of the dominant follicle. Furthermore, ultrasonography permits follow-up of the growth velocity of the leading follicle, to determine complete follicular maturity and

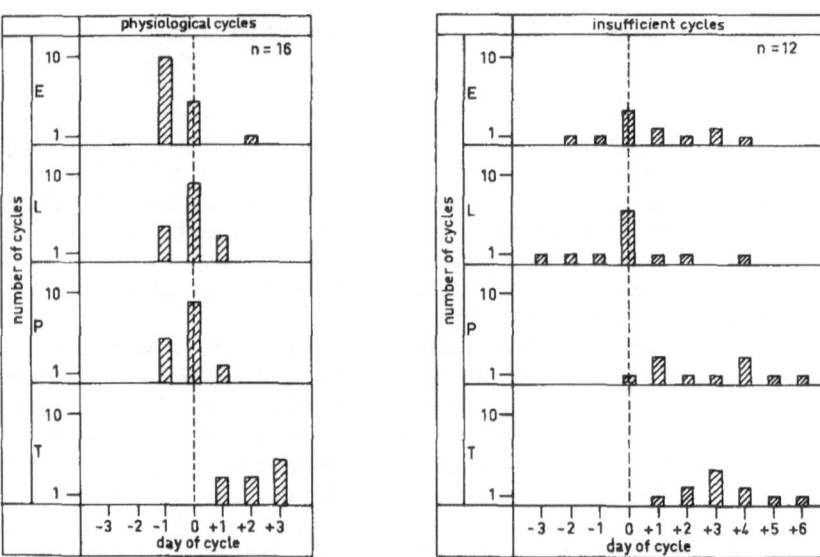

Figure 8.6 Comparison of endocrinological findings between apparently normal and insufficient cycles

to predict ovulation. In addition, it is possible to monitor the development of the corpus luteum with its various forms as solid or cystic structures.

Furthermore, insufficient cycles can be monitored by this technique and the findings can be correlated to endocrinological data. Summarizing the results presented, we conclude that an inadequate luteal function can be regarded as a consequence of impaired follicular development being characterized as disturbed selection and maturation of the leading follicle.

References

1. Tredway, D. R., Mishell, D. R. and Moyer, D. L. (1973). Correlation of endometrial dating with luteinizing hormone peak. *Am. J. Obstet. Gynecol.*, **117**, 1030
2. Wentz, A. C. (1980). Endometrial biopsy in the evaluation of infertility. *Fertil. Steril.*, **33**, 121
3. Sherman, B. M. and Korenman, S. G. (1974). Measurement of plasma LH, FSH, estradiol and progesterone in disorders of the human menstrual cycle: the short luteal phase. *J. Clin. Endocrinol. Metab.*, **38**, 89
4. Sherman, B. M. and Korenman, S. G. (1974). Measurement of serum LH, FSH, estradiol and progesterone in disorders of the human menstrual cycle: the inadequate luteal phase. *J. Clin. Endocrinol. Metab.*, **39**, 145
5. Stouffer, R. L. and Hodgen, G. D. (1980). Induction of luteal phase defects in rhesus monkeys by follicular fluid administration at onset of the menstrual cycle. *J. Clin. Endocrinol. Metab.*, **51**, 669
6. McNatty, K. P., Smith, D. M., Makris, A., Osathanondh, R. R. and Ryan, K. J. (1979). The microenvironment of the human antral follicles: interrelationship among the steroid levels in antral fluid, the population of granulosa cells and status of the oocyte *in vivo* and *in vitro*. *J. Clin. Endocrinol. Metab.*, **49**, 851
7. Di Zerega, G. S. and Hodgen, G. D. (1981). Luteal phase dysfunction infertility: a sequel to aberrant folliculogenesis. *Fertil. Steril.*, **35**, 489
8. Geisthövel, F., Skubsch, U., Zabel, G., Schillinger, H. and Breckwoldt, M. (1983). Ultrasonographic and hormonal studies in physiological and insufficient menstrual cycles. *Fertil. Steril.*, **39**, 277
9. Hackelöer, B. J., Fleming, R., Robinson, H. P., Adam, A. H. and Couts, J. R. T. (1979). Correlation of ultrasonic and endocrinologic assessment of human follicular development. *Am. J. Obstet. Gynecol.*, **135**, 122
10. Polan, M. L., Totora, M., Caldwell, B. V., De Cherney, A. H., Haseltine, F. P. and Kase, N. (1982). Abnormal ovarian cycles as diagnosed by ultrasound and serum estradiol levels. *Fertil. Steril.*, **37**, 342
11. Renaud, R. L., Mader, J., Dervain, J., Ehret, M.-C., Aron, C., Plasa-Roser, S., Spira, A. and Pollack, H. (1980). Echographic study of follicular maturation and ovulation during the normal menstrual cycle. *Fertil. Steril.*, **33**, 272

Discussion

Rothchild	What seems to be the luteinization of an atretic follicle is extremely interesting as there is a parallel to some experiments done in rats, in which by delaying the LH-surge with barbiturate administration in the pre-estrus for 2 or 3 days, the hormonal picture changes remarkably, as there is a drop in estrogen and androgen production, and an increase in progesterone secretion. It is the increased pattern of progesterone secretion which is identical to what we would call in the human being an ICL. It never gets to the level that is characteristic of the normal corpus luteum. The luteinized theca cells have been identified as being the source of this progesterone secretion. I wonder if you have any thoughts on this subject? What is happening in these atretic follicles is not the luteinization of the granulosa cells, because the characteristic of atresia is that the granulosa cells disappear. This may be one of the important forms of what we call an ICL. It is really not a ruptured follicle that is luteinized partially, but an atretic follicle in which the theca is luteinized to produce enough progesterone to look like a luteal phase.
Insler	I have to confess that we are unable to measure with any certainty follicles of 10 mm in diameter or less. We therefore cannot be certain that we are following the same follicle if it does not grow beyond 12–13 mm.
Breckwoldt	It depends a little on the equipment that is available and to a large degree on the man who uses it. Franz Geisthövel has become a real expert, and he may give you some detailed information on the equipment and techniques he uses.
Insler	I found it extremely interesting that there was a large cystic structure at the beginning of the cycle in one or both ovaries in those cycles which were finally diagnosed as insufficient. This would actually be another proof for the assumption that the biological clock is entirely in the ovary, and that the cycle does not begin during menstruation but a few days earlier. The fate of the cycle is really determined during the preceding corpus luteum phase.
Runnebaum	It is very important to have ultrasound in order to recognize the stage at which the selection of the dominant follicle occurs. How important is it, however, to have in addition each day a determination of estradiol for the purpose of correlation? Is there a correlation between the ultrasound findings and the estradiol levels when the dominant follicle undergoes atresia and does not attain the stage of ovulation?
Breckwoldt	I think it is most important to have daily monitoring in the critical phase during which selection occurs. If you take a blood sample, e.g. on a Sunday, you will not obtain a result, and you will have to rely on your sonographic findings. It is difficult to discriminate between insufficient and physiological cycles by means of the estradiol production.
Runnebaum	Sometimes the follicle does not grow any further even though the estrogens continue to rise, eventually to a level of 1500 pg/ml or more. What happens to such a follicle?
Breckwoldt	There must be growth of a follicle when the estradiol levels increase, as it has to mature to produce such large amounts of estrogen.

Bettendorf	We have also seen the reverse, a growing follicle without a simultaneous rise in serum estradiol. This occurs quite often during stimulation therapy.
Geisthövel	Another type of insufficient cycle is that with follicular persistence. We observed acyclic follicular persistence with estradiol levels below 100 pg/ml in one patient.
Keller	These data are very fascinating but what do they mean clinically with respect to treatment? You made the statement that the fate of the cycle is decided very early. Did you consequently stop using any stimulation or supplementation therapy in the second half of the cycle?
Breckwoldt	Well, I think we should leave this point to the discussion of the therapeutic aspects, but I think that we should stimulate the follicle during follicular development.
Daume	What you said about the development and disappearance of cystic follicles was very important. They may appear with or without luteinization. If luteinization takes place, there is no chance for ovulation to occur during this cycle. If the cystic structures come and go, and there is no luteinization, it is possible to succeed in inducing ovulation at a very late time of the cycle, e.g. day 18–20, by stimulation therapy. At least one clinical parameter should be included into the monitoring, preferably the cervical score. When the score increases, estrogens should be determined, and one should have the possibility of obtaining a rapid estimate of progesterone if the score indicates that ovulation may have taken place.
Breckwoldt	In daily practice, we see the patients, check the cervical score according to Insler *et al.* (*Int. J. Gynecol. Obstet.*, **10**, (1972), 200) and, when the secretion has increased, tell the patient that the selection of the follicle has occurred, and she should now also be subjected to ultrasound.
Wentz	Looking at these cycles it appeared that you had cycles of varying follicular length and variable luteal length, and variable total length, which again takes me back to considering what the patient population was to begin with, and how you defined the inadequate cycle. The question that follows on that is, under what circumstances, or how many times, were you able to follow a patient sequentially such that you were able to determine that this patient indeed had repetitive LPI, and not a situation in which you just happened to pick up an abnormal cycle, that, we all agree, would not require treatment?
Breckwoldt	The length of the cycle and of the follicular phase is variable but that of the luteal phase is rather constant, i.e. 14 days, maximally 16 days. Such cycles were defined as being apparently normal. In this study we did not follow patients in successive cycles. The cycles were defined according to the length of the whole cycle and that of the luteal phase, and on the basis of progesterone measurements done during the latter. The only variable was the length of the selection phase, while you see all these small follicles. The time that elapses from selection to full maturation is again rather constant, 5–7 days.
Bettendorf	This is in good agreement with data we have from hMG therapy.
Wentz	I would like to make a comment with respect to endometrial height. We have obviously been most interested in endometrial height in patients who have been monitored both in normal and in clomid-stimulated cycles and in hMG-induced cycles. I wonder if you found what we have in comparing these three groups of patients? As everyone knows, in clomid-stimulated patients who are allowed to ovulate without hCG, a peak estradiol level will be achieved that is equal to about 500 pg/ml times the number of dominant follicles as seen by ultrasound. In our patients induced by clomid we may see a peak estradiol between 1000 and 1500 pg/ml. In our hMG-stimulated cycles we ordinarily do not let these individuals get quite to the same levels at the time we give hCG. The interesting phenomenon that I will be happy to have you comment upon, is the finding of endometrial height. In clomid-treated patients whose estradiol level was in the 1500 pg/ml range

111

compared to hMG-treated patients whose estradiol was perhaps in the 500 pg/ml range, there is an inverse proportion of height of the endometrium. We have found that those individuals who have the highest estradiol levels if they are clomid-treated, have an endometrial height of approximately one-third to one-half that of hMG-treated patients. I wonder if you would agree that perhaps this is a reflection of the anti-estrogenic effect of clomid?

Breckwoldt   There seem to be certain limitations to respond to these estrogen levels. We have done experiments on cell cultures where the endometrial cells were exposed to various levels of estrogen, and the incorporation of [^{3}H]thymidine was measured. We noted that the incorporation would increase to a certain level, but it would decrease again when the estrogens were raised beyond a threshold. This means that the activity of the endometrium would be inhibited. There is something like a physiological range of estrogens the endometrium may be exposed to. The anti-estrogenic effect may explain this phenomenon, but I am not sure about that. Both the pharmacological effect of the circulating estrogens and the anti-estrogenic effect of clomiphene may act in concert upon the endometrium, and this may result in a reduced endometrial height.

9
The diagnostic value of the endometrial biopsy

J. P. VIELH, J. DE BRUX, K. NAHOUL AND J. P. GAUTRAY

The concept of luteal insufficiency was first proposed by G. S. Jones[1], who used endometrial biopsies (EB) as an estimate of the hormonal balance in disorders of the menstrual cycle. Its value was recently re-emphasized by the same author[2,3]. Since hormonal measurements have become easier and more precise, the respective values of hormonal evaluations and the EB have become a matter of debate[4-6]. Many endocrinologists are not accustomed to perform and interpret EB, and rather rely on hormonal measurements[7-11]. The physiological and clinical importance of correlating different clinical parameters such as the basal body-temperature chart, hormonal measurements, and the EB has been demonstrated by Taubert[12]. The aim of this study was to set forth the informational quality of the EB – provided the histological readings are carried out with care and precision; and to correlate the EB and hormonal measurements for a better understanding of the physiopathology of the menstrual cycle.

MATERIAL AND METHODS

Histological patterns

The histological basis of the evaluation of the endometrium has been precisely defined by Noyes et al.[13-15]. As the hormonal influences occurring during the ovarian cycle correspond to clearly recognizable histological patterns, dating of the endometrium to the nearest possible day becomes feasible by comparison with a factual or assumed 28-day cycle. Even though this type of evaluation can reach a high level of precision, not infrequently, histological reports allow only a rough estimate of the situation. Six characteristic elements should be taken into account for a clear evaluation of endometrial histology; the first three are:

(1) glandular mitoses and pseudostratification of the nuclei (both being characteristic of the proliferative phase);

(2) basal vacuolization (earliest morphological evidence of ovulation according to Noyes *et al.*[13], and of the influence of progesterone according to de Brux);

(3) secretory changes, presence of stromal mitoses, and of leucocytic infiltration.

In our opinion, three other parameters should also be considered:

(4) the development of the spiral arteries is usually in concordance with the actual day of the cycle, and facilitates the dating of the endometrium;

(5) the significance of the total thickness of the endometrium has already been pointed out by Noyes[16]; it is seldom taken into account, although it presents valuable evidence of the estrogen secretion during the follicular phase;

(6) distended or cystic endometrial glands appear to be related to a steep decrease of progesterone secretion.

There are two predominant histological patterns in luteal defect:

(1) *maturative delay* is a more than 2 days lag in the effect of progesterone upon the endometrium as compared to the secretory change seen on the same day of a 28-day reference cycle;

(2) the same type of abnormality may be associated with a dystrophic pattern such as *persistent mitoses in the glandular epithelium*. This provides evidence that the estrogenic influence is persistent, and has not been blocked by progesterone[17, 18].

The EB should be performed at a proper time of the cycle to demonstrate these histological patterns in a case of luteal defect. The day 21 to day 23 period has been chosen for three reasons in our study:

(1) it corresponds to the zenith of corpus luteum activity, during which the imprint of progesterone action occurs;

(2) during that period the endometrium has completed its necessary transformation for ovum implantation to occur;

(3) when the EB is performed later in the cycle, the premenstrual changes of the endometrium, e.g. diffusion by blood etc., may interfere with an accurate histological interpretation.

Between 1 July 1982, and 30 June 1983, 174 EB have been performed by our clinical group according to the same protocol; the histological interpretation of the specimen was always done by the same pathologist (J. de Brux).

Endocrine parameters

A correlative study was attempted, to compare the histological findings both as to length and balance of the two phases of the cycle[19], and the results of the hormone measurements.

In clinical practice it is quite impossible to obtain daily measurements of gonadotropins and of steroids, or to repeat biopsies. For that reason a

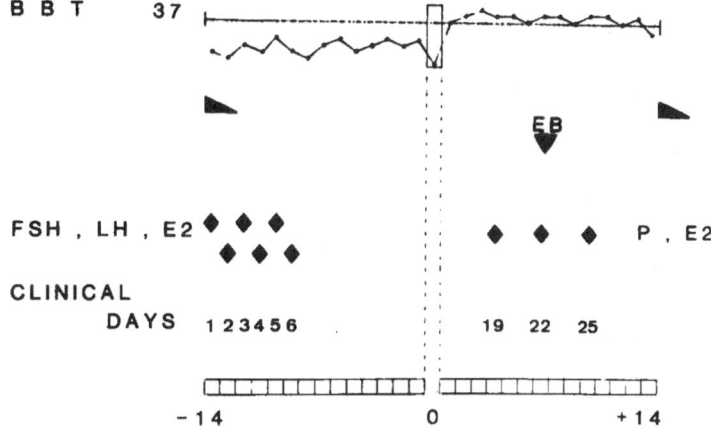

Figure 9.1 Diagrammatic representation of the protocol for the investigation of the menstrual cycle. 0 = Day of ovulation; EB = endometrial biopsy

protocol of investigation was designed to obtain as much information as possible with the least amount of disturbance (Figure 9.1).

(1) The basal body-temperature chart is used to estimate the date of ovulation, and that day is considered as Day 0. Consequently, the days of the follicular days are referred to as Day −1, −2 etc., and the days of the luteal phase as Day 1, 2 etc.

(2) During the early follicular phase (1st week of the cycle), three measurements of LH, FSH, and estradiol are performed, as an endocrine imbalance during this period of the cycle may induce disorders in both the granulosa cell maturation, and the luteal phase[21–24].

(3) Three measurements of progesterone and estradiol are done on Day 19, 22, and 25 for a statistically valid evaluation of corpus luteum secretory function, as three normal values of progesterone have been reported[25] as being indicative of luteal phase adequacy. All measurements were performed by using appropriate radioimmunoassays[26–28].

Between July 1982 and June 1983, 148 cycles have been investigated according to this protocol. The results have not been published elsewhere.

RESULTS AND DISCUSSION

Statistical data are deliberately not presented, but several characteristic cases will be discussed as a basis for physiopathological reflection.

Endometrial biopsies and hormone measurements are in agreement

The data obtained in a normal cycle are presented in Figure 9.2. The infertility of this patient was caused by tubal occlusion. The hormone measurements are within the limits of the norm, and the EB revealed a normal secretory

115

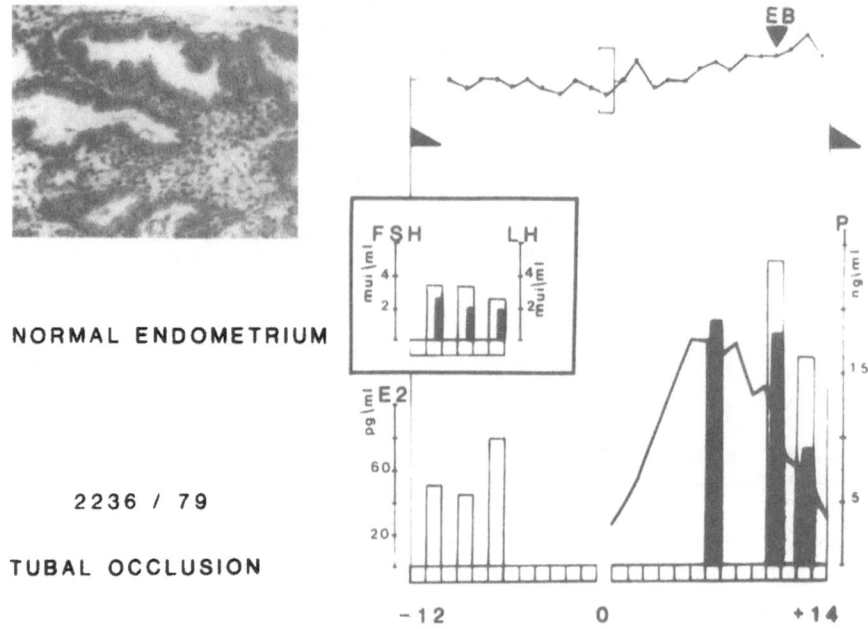

NORMAL ENDOMETRIUM

2236 / 79

TUBAL OCCLUSION

Figure 9.2 Normal menstrual cycle: The infecundity is due to tubal occlusion. Open bars: estradiol; solid bars: progesterone; endometrium: normal secretory transformation

endometrium. Figure 9.3 also represents data of a cycle which must be considered as normal, since the patient conceived. The endometrium is perfectly in-phase, and the values of serum progesterone are rather high.

Two types of luteal defect have previously been described[17],

(1) the pure luteal defect (LD), and
(2) the luteal defect with persistent estrogenic influence (LD + PEI), and a correlation between the result of the EB and of the hormone measurements could be shown. The hormonal disturbance is more severe in LD + PEI.

Reduced thickness of the endometrium is characteristic of estrogenic insufficiency during the follicular phase. In these cases, the thickness mean value was $120\,\mu m$ instead of $180-200\,\mu m$, i.e. a 30% reduction. This may, however, be the only endometrial abnormality, the other histological features being normal, as if the periovulatory phase was hormonally inconspicuous. Nevertheless, a luteal defect can be observed in such a situation.

It should be pointed out that in all normal or disturbed cycles there was a good correlation between the results of the endometrial biopsy and the hormonal evaluations.

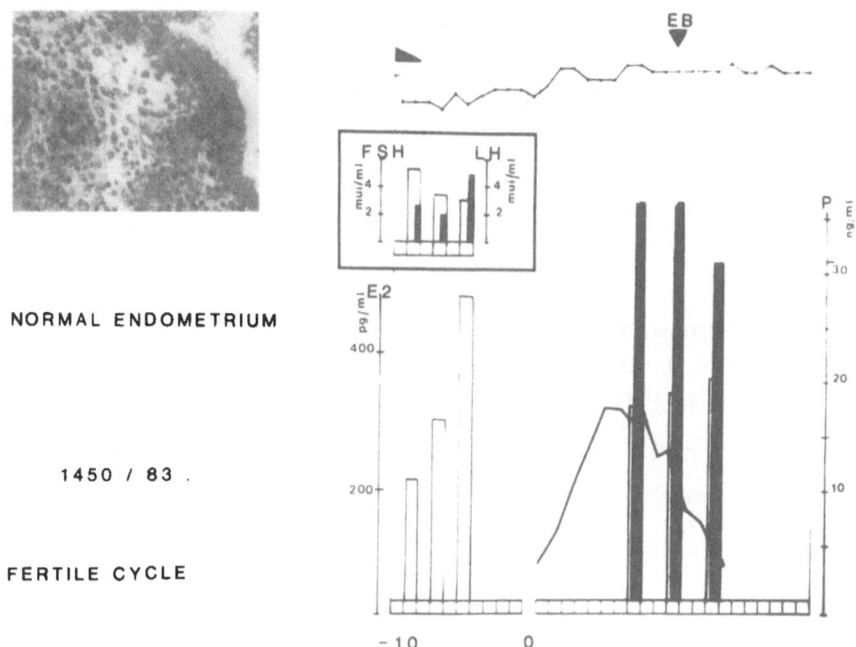

NORMAL ENDOMETRIUM

1450 / 83 .

FERTILE CYCLE

Figure 9.3 Fertile cycle. Endometrium: normal secretory transformation. Open bars: E₂; solid bars: P

Endometrial biopsies and hormone measurements are not in agreement

Patients with a *short follicular phase* are a first group in this category requiring attention. The proposed method of investigation may suggest what appears to be a dissociation between the EB and the hormone values, when ovulation occurs earlier than usual. This phenomenon may not be pathological in that the EB is in phase and the hormone values are normal for the end of the cycle which can be ascertained by the basal body-temperature record. As the effect of progesterone on the secretion has been normal during the early luteal phase, short follicular phases may occur during abnormal cycles, too. In the case shown in Figure 9.4, the endometrium is almost normal, but the glandular tubules are cystic. Moreover the hormone values, although determined somewhat late in the cycle, demonstrate luteal insufficiency. This type of data certainly invites some speculation. The immediate preovulatory period has probably been normal with respect to the induction of endometrial progesterone receptors, and a short-lasting progesterone secretion has been sufficient to determine a luteal endometrial pattern. Such a short-lasting progesterone secretion may not be infrequent in unexplained infertility, but can only be demonstrated by frequent measurements, and a careful correlative study of all cycle parameters.

117

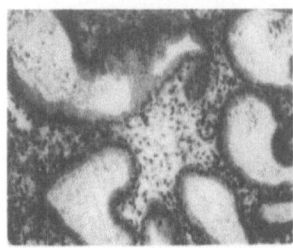

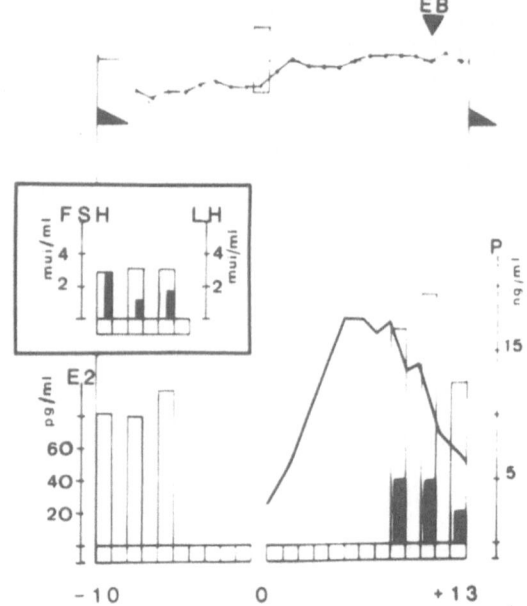

NORMAL ENDOMETRIUM
BUT DILATED TUBES
EARLY OVULATION

1701 / 82

LUTEAL DEFECT

Figure 9.4 Infecundity due to luteal defect. The whole cycle is abnormal: early ovulation, probably anomaly of the endometrium (see text), and obvious luteal insufficiency. Open bars: E₂; solid bars: P

Women with a *short luteal phase* represent another important group. The differences between the EB and hormone levels cannot be attributed any longer to the protocol of investigation, but to a functional disorder of the cycle induced by a kinetic abnormality of hormonal secretion. In such a situation the EB may be normal and misleading, as the abnormality is due to a short life-span of the corpus luteum. If the progesterone secretion has been adequate during the period when the endometrial progesterone receptors are physiologically receptive, the endometrium may be in phase, and the disorder can only be ascertained by the basal body-temperature record and hormone measurements. The short luteal phase may be characterized by the following findings:

(1) In the first category, both EB and hormone levels are normal, but the corpus luteum lifespan is too short, and this can be demonstrated by BBT charts.

(2) In another group the EB is normal, but the disturbance can be ascertained by both the basal body-temperature record and hormone levels.

(3) In a third group of cases the EB also appears to be in phase, but an initially high progesterone secretion is followed by a steep decrease to low levels; in this type of case the endometrial glands may appear cystic.

It is our opinion that these three examples not only illustrate possibly distinct classes of luteal defect, but also re-emphasize the diagnostic value of the EB.

CONCLUSIONS

(1) A single endometrial sample is sufficient for such an investigation as it renders global but precise information, and mirrors the endocrine and/or histological events occurring during the preceding 22 or 23 days of the cycle.

(2) The informational value of the EB depends on a detailed histological report which must follow several well-defined criteria.

(3) The EB is the only method which can also demonstrate other endometrial lesions, such as endometritis.

Differences between the EB and hormone measurements should not lead to giving an advantage to either method, as normal secretory transformation of the endometrium can be observed in the presence of decreased levels of progesterone and estradiol in serum and vice-versa. These facts should lead to a debate on the temporal and kinetic evolution of normal hormone concentrations, and on the capacity and conditions of endometrial receptivity. These reflections should be of help in understanding as yet unexplained cases of infertility.

References

1. Jones, G. S. (1949). Some newer aspects of the management of infertility. *J. Am. Med. Assoc.*, **141**, 1123
2. Moszowski, E., Woodruff, J. D. and Jones, G. E. S. (1962). The inadequate luteal phase. *Am. J. Obstet. Gynecol.*, **83**, 363
3. Jones, G. S. (1976). The luteal phase defect. *Fertil. Steril.*, **27**, 351
4. Rosenfeld, D. L. and Garcia, C. R. (1976). A comparison of endometrial histology with simultaneous plasma progesterone determination of infertile women. *Fertil. Steril.*, **27**, 1256
5. Wentz, A. C. (1982). Diagnosing luteal phase inadequacy. *Fertil. Steril.*, **37**, 334
6. Abdulla, V., Diver, M. J., Hipkin, L. J. and David, J. C. (1983). Plasma progesterone levels as an index of ovulation. *Br. J. Obstet. Gynaecol.*, **90**, 543
7. Strott, C. A., Cargille, C. M., Ross, G. T. and Lipsett, M. B. (1970). The short luteal phase. *J. Clin. Endocrinol. Metab.*, **30**, 246
8. Sherman, B. M. and Korenman, S. G. (1974). Measurement of plasma LH, FSH, estradiol and progesterone in disorders of the human menstrual cycle: the short luteal phase. *J. Clin. Endocrinol. Metab.*, **38**, 89
9. Sherman, B. M. and Korenman, S. G. (1974). Measurement of serum LH, FSH, estradiol and progesterone in disorders of the human menstrual cycle: the inadequate luteal phase. *J. Clin. Endocrinol. Metab.*, **39**, 145
10. Wilks, J. W., Hodgen, G. D. and Ross, G. T. (1976). Luteal phase defects in the rhesus monkey: the significance of serum FSH:LH ratios. *J. Clin. Endocrinol. Metab.*, **43**, 1261
11. Nass, T. E., Dierschke, D. J., Clerk, J. R., Meller, P. A. and Schillo, K. K. (1979). Luteal phase deficiencies in peripubertal rhesus monkey: mechanistic considerations. In Channing, C. P., Marsh, J. and Sadler, W. A. (eds.) *Ovarian Follicular and Corpus Luteum Function.* p. 519. (New York: Plenum Press)
12. Taubert, H. D. (1978). Luteal phase insufficiency. In Keller, J. P. (ed.) *Female Infertility.* pp. 78–113. (Basel: Karger)
13. Noyes, R. W., Hertig, A. T. and Rock, J. (1950). Dating the endometrial biopsy. *Fertil. Steril.*, **1**, 3
14. Noyes, R. W. and Haman, J. O. (1953). The accuracy of endometrial dating. *Fertil. Steril.*, **4**, 504

15. Noyes, R. W. (1966). Endometrial dating for the detection of ovulation. In Greenblatt, R. B. (ed.) *Ovulation*. pp. 319–328. (Philadelphia: Lippincott)
16. Noyes, R. W. (1959). The underdeveloped secretory endometrium. *Am. J. Obstet. Gynecol.*, **77**, 929
17. Gautray, J. P., de Brux, J., Tajchner, G., Robel, P. and Mouren, M. (1981). Clinical investigation of the menstrual cycle. III. Clinical, endometrial, and endocrine aspects of luteal defect. *Fertil. Steril.*, **35**, 296
18. de Brux, J. Evaluation of ovarian disturbances by endometrial biopsy. In de Brux, J., Mortel, R. and Gautray, J. P. (eds.) *The Endometrium: Hormonal Impacts*. Volume 1, pp. 107–122. (New York: Plenum Press)
19. Jolivet, A. and Gautray, J. P. (1978). Clinical investigation of the menstrual cycle. I. Diagram of the normal menstrual cycle. *Fertil. Steril.*, **29**, 40
20. Wilks, J. W., Hodgen, G. D. and Ross, G. T. (1977). Anovulatory menstrual cycles in the rhesus monkey: the significance of serum FSH/LH ratios. *Fertil. Steril.*, **28**, 1094
21. Stouffer, R. L. and Hodgen, G. D. (1980). Induction of luteal phase defects in rhesus monkey by follicular fluid administration at the onset of the menstrual cycle. *J. Clin. Endocrinol. Metab.*, **51**, 669
22. Richards, J. S. and Bogovich, K. (1980). Development of gonadotrophin receptors during follicular growth. In Mahesh, V. B., Muldoon, T. G., Saxena, B. B. and Sadler, W. A. (eds.) *Functional Correlates of Hormone Receptors in Reproduction*. pp. 223–244. (Amsterdam: Elsevier North Holland)
23. Di Zerega, G. S. and Hodgen, G. D. (1981). Follicular phase treatment of luteal phase dysfunction. *Fertil. Steril.*, **35**, 428
24. Di Zerega, G. S. and Hodgen, G. D. (1981). Luteal phase dysfunction infertility: a sequel to aberrant folliculogenesis. *Fertil. Steril.*, **35**, 489
25. Scholler, R., Nahoul, K. and Blacker, C. (1981). Biochemical evaluation of corpus luteum function. In de Brux, J., Mortel, R. and Gautray, J. P. (eds.) *The Endometrium: Hormonal Impacts*. pp. 81–106. (New York: Plenum Press)
26. Castanier, M. and Scholler, R. (1970). Dosage radio-immunologique de l'estrone et de l'estradiol-17 beta plasmatiques. *C.R. Acad. Sci. Paris*, **271**, 1787
27. Roger, M., Veinante, A., Soldat, M. C., Tardy, J., Tribondeau, E. and Scholler, R. (1975). Etude simultanée des gonadotrophines, des oestrogènes, de la progestérone et de la 17-hydroxyprogestérone plasmatiques au cours du cycle ovulatoire. *Nouv. Presse Méd.*, **4**, 2173
28. Tea, N. T., Castanier, M., Roger, M. and Scholler, R. (1975). Simultaneous radioimmunoassay of plasma progesterone and 17α-hydroxyprogesterone. Normal values in children, in men and in women throughout the menstrual cycle and in early pregnancy. *J. Steroid Biochem.*, **6**, 1509

Discussion

Dallenbach-Hellweg	I do not think that day 21–23 of the cycle is the ideal time for endometrial biopsy, as you may overlook important changes in the endometrial stroma which occur only during the second part of the luteal phase. Progesterone acts first on the glandular epithelial cells. Thereafter, i.e. after 7 days, it begins to have an effect upon the stromal cells, and brings about predecidual and granulocytic differentiation. These changes are as important as those in the glandular cells, but you can consider and evaluate them only during the late luteal phase. As a consequence, the ideal time for an endometrial biopsy is the late secretory phase, but not before day 26 of a 28-day cycle.
	The so-called regressive changes that you mentioned do not really occur in the endometrium before menstruation starts. There is a decrease in endometrial height due to fluid loss, but there are no degenerative changes in the endometrial stroma noticeable until menstruation ensues.
Gautray	There is a histological basis that we take the samples earlier in the cycle in that this phase is probably more in accordance with chemical modifications of the endometrium, receptor values, and enzymatic variations with respect to nidation.
Taubert	We used to do biopsies on or about day 21 of the cycle, but we dropped this approach and chose to follow the method described by Dr Dallenbach, as it is extremely difficult to select the proper day on the basis of the basal temperature record when a biopsy is to be performed during the mid-luteal phase. It has been pointed out rightly that it is very difficult to obtain daily measurements of estradiol and of LH in clinical practice. We therefore took a different approach and asked patients to save daily morning-urine specimens from day 5 of the cycle until 2–3 days after the expected time of ovulation. Even though our experience is limited as yet, we found it possible to delineate the LH-peak in a more or less pronounced manner, and to use this information for timing ovulation. My question is, have you had any experience with this type of approach?
Gautray	Not with the type of procedure which you showed on your slide.
Lehmann	In the last three examples you demonstrated there was a problem in that you did not indicate the day of ovulation but by counting the days of the basal temperature record. If you would allow just an error of 2–3 days to the left of the chart, you would find the endometrium to be completely in-phase. All the other parameters shown on the graph were normal, only the count of the days did not fit.
Gautray	I do not think we are always in-phase, we are more frequently out-of-phase, if we do not appreciate and choose the day of biopsy carefully.
Lehmann	Out-of-phase by what? By counting the days or by endometrial dating?
Gautray	By endometrial dating according to the criteria established by Noyes *et al.* (*Fertil Steril.*, 1 (1950), 3).
Lehmann	I do not doubt your capability to date the endometrium. I just say that counting the days of the cycle does not necessarily yield information which fits to what is happening physiologically.

Rothchild   One of the big problems with such an attempt at correlating endocrine and endometrial parameters with the time of ovulation is the use of the basal temperature record as the source of information. It is a perfectly good reflection of the effect of progesterone on the regulation of body temperature control mechanisms, but the time of the shift of the body temperature is not absolutely correlated with the progesterone secretion rise. It was pointed out 20 years ago that there may be as much as a 3-day difference between the time that temperature changes and the time ovulation actually occurred, as determined by actual observation of the ovary at laparotomy. So one needs a more exact indicator of the time of ovulation. The basal body temperature can be a useful indicator as to when to focus down to get exact information, but by itself it may lead to the sort of discrepancy we are talking about.

Gautray   It is true that it is a clinical investigative tool. The reported cases are taken from the files of a sterility clinic, they do not reflect normal physiological circumstances. These individuals were not volunteers.

Rothchild   You need something more exact, like a radioreceptor assay for the LH peak. That would give you a much more precise time of ovulation.

Gautray   This would require one or even more than one determination per day, and this is difficult to carry out in the setting of a sterility clinic.

Wentz   I simply wanted to say what essentially has been said. We all review the literature, and in *Fertility and Sterility* in the last 18 months there have been no fewer than six articles which have taken either LH-peaks, the BBT, or ultrasound criteria, and have shown the exceedingly poor ability to use the BBT to what you are doing. In fact, if you simply turn that slide on again (Figure 9.4), it will become apparent that it will be very difficult to pick where you would date ovulation. But even more important are data which suggest that taking the biopsy does not accelerate the onset of menses, and for this reason we have used the time of the onset of bleeding as a marker to date our endometriums. I would think it would be exceedingly beneficial to go back over your endometrium which is impeccably dated and diagnosed, but using the criteria of when the biopsy was taken with respect to when menses occurred, and to see whether you had under those circumstances a different correlation, or the same correlation. If then you could show that you were able to do exactly what could be done by dating backwards, then I would agree completely and think that this would be a perfectly acceptable time.

10
Evaluation of luteal insufficiency by hormone load tests

I. GERHARD AND B. RUNNEBAUM

Though evidence of ovulation can be obtained by a single serum progesterone (P) assay, controversial views on the necessity of serial P determinations or endometrial biopsies for confirmation of luteal phase adequacy continue to exist[1-11]. Due to the short biological half-life of P the single determination affords only a vague insight into the corpus luteum function[2, 12-15].

In vitro and *in vivo* P production by the corpus luteum can be stimulated by the LH releasing hormone (LH-RH), luteinizing hormone (LH) and human chorionic gonadotropin (hCG)[16-20]. On the other hand, functional disorders of other endocrine organs, such as hyperprolactinaemia, hyperandrogenaemia and diseases of the thyroid gland, can suppress the corpus luteum function[21-23].

It is also likely that an assessment of the corpus luteum function is possible through other steroids as well, such as estradiol-17β (E$_2$) or 17α-hydroxyprogesterone (17-OHP)[24]. As there is no binding definition for corpus luteum insufficiency, the following studies examine further assessment of the corpus luteum function through stimulation tests.

hCG TEST

Our study comprises 76 women who complained of infertility. The basal body temperature charts (BBT) showed ovulation between days 6 and 24 with a raised temperature for periods of 11–16 days. The basal concentrations of FSH, LH, prolactin, testosterone, dehydroepiandrosterone sulphate, T$_3$, T$_4$ and TSH were normal.

The women were hospitalized between days 5 and 8 of the hyperthermic phase, and the cubital vein was catheterized for blood sampling. The patients were randomly divided into four groups of 19 women each who received intramuscular injections of $10/20/40 \times 1000$ IU hCG or physiologic saline. Blood samples were taken every 3 h over a 24 h period, and then every second day until onset of menstruation. All samples of one patient were run in the same assay. The serum concentrations of β-hCG, prolactin, P, 17-OHP, and E₂ were radioimmunologically determined.

The assays were carried out with specific antibodies as previously described[20]. The following characteristics of each hormone response curve were stored in the computer program and are given in Figure 10.1. These parameters were correlated to one another and to clinical items by means of the χ^2, Friedman, Wilcoxon, and Kruskal–Wallis tests and Spearman correlation coefficients. The level of significance was chosen for $p < 0.01$.

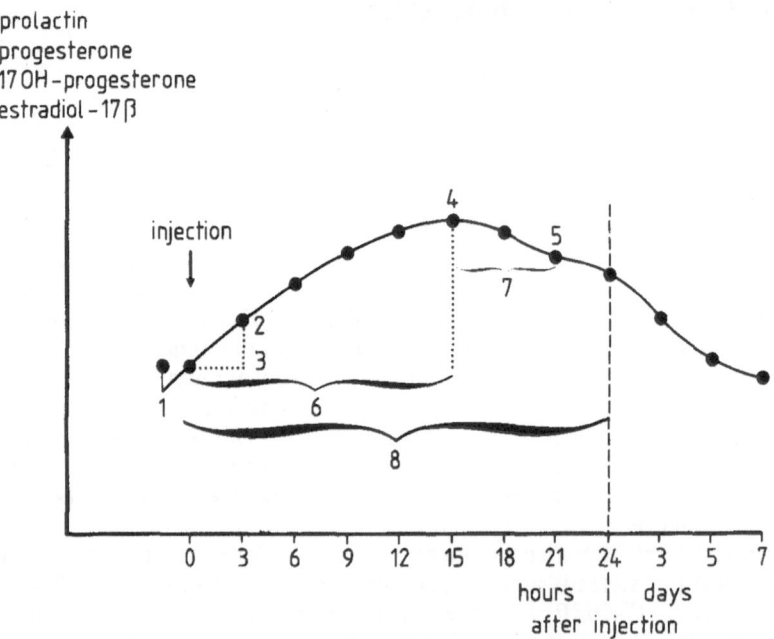

Figure 10.1 Characteristics of the hormone response curves following intramuscular (i.m.) injection of hCG. Times of blood sampling are indicated on the abscissa: (1) base value (base val); (2) net increase for each interval (net inc); (3) percentage increase for each interval (% inc); (4) maximum within 24 h (max); (5) minimum within 24 h (min); (6) time needed for max. increase (*t* max); (7) time needed for 20% decrease of max. value (*t* min); (8) area below the curve over 24 h; (9) max, min and area of the net inc and of the percentage inc

The clinical data of the four groups of patients tested are summarized in Tables 10.1 and 10.2. The medians of each group are also given. Statistical evaluation proved that none of the items differed significantly, so that the results of the individual hCG doses may well be compared to each other.

The β-hCG-concentrations showed significant dose-dependent increases in all patients up to 24 h after injection (Figure 10.2). Dose-dependency could be demonstrated up to the menstrual period.

The E₂ concentrations exhibited a significant circadian rhythm after injections of physiologic saline with decreasing values over the day and

Table 10.1   Clinical data I of 76 women with hormone load tests during the luteal phase

Items (median)	Physiologic saline (n = 19)	10 000 IU hCG (n = 19)	20 000 IU hCG (n = 19)	40 000 IU hCG (n = 19)
Age (years)	29	28	27	32
Weight (kg)	56	57	56	59
Height (cm)	168	164	170	164
Duration of infertility (years)	4	4	4	5
No. of pregnancies after testing	8	9	9	8

Table 10.2   Clinical data II of 76 women with hormone load tests during the luteal phase

Items (median)	Physiologic saline (n = 19)	10 000 IU hCG (n = 19)	20 000 IU hCG (n = 19)	40 000 IU hCG (n = 19)
Menarche (years)	13	13	13	13
Day of ovulation	15	15	16	15
Duration of luteal phase (days)	12	13	13	13
Basal values				
Prolactin (ng/ml)	13	14	13	14
Progesterone (ng/ml)	10	12	13	11
17-OH-Progesterone (ng/ml)	5	4	4	6
Estradiol-17β (pg/ml)	151	151	161	195

increasing concentrations in the evening (9 and 12 p.m.) (Figure 10.3). At all intervals examined results of the hCG tests were significantly different from those of the placebo group. The hCG injections effected a continuous level of diurnal E_2 concentrations. A more distinct increase was observed in the evening. E_2 concentrations declined below the basal values 24 h after injection; 3 and 5 days after injection the E_2 concentrations had reached a significantly higher level as compared to that before injection. Not until 7 days after the injection significant differences between the individual hCG doses could be observed. The E_2 concentrations after 40 000 IU hCG showed a marked increase as compared to the values after 10 and 20×1000 IU.

P concentrations of the placebo group also showed a significant diurnal rhythm with decreasing values over the day and an increase in the evening. Peaks were observed at night and towards the morning (Figure 10.4). At all time intervals the placebo group showed significantly different values compared to the hCG test groups. The hCG injections led to a double peak P secretion with the first peak observed after approximately 12 h and a second, much more pronounced one, after 3 and 5 days. The absolute P values showed no differences between the individual dosage levels; 15, 18 and 21 h following injection the net and percentage increases however, showed a peak after 10 000 IU hCG and reached their lowest level after 20 000 IU hCG. Seven days following injection P concentrations were significantly higher after 20 and 40×1000 IU hCG than after 10 000 IU hCG.

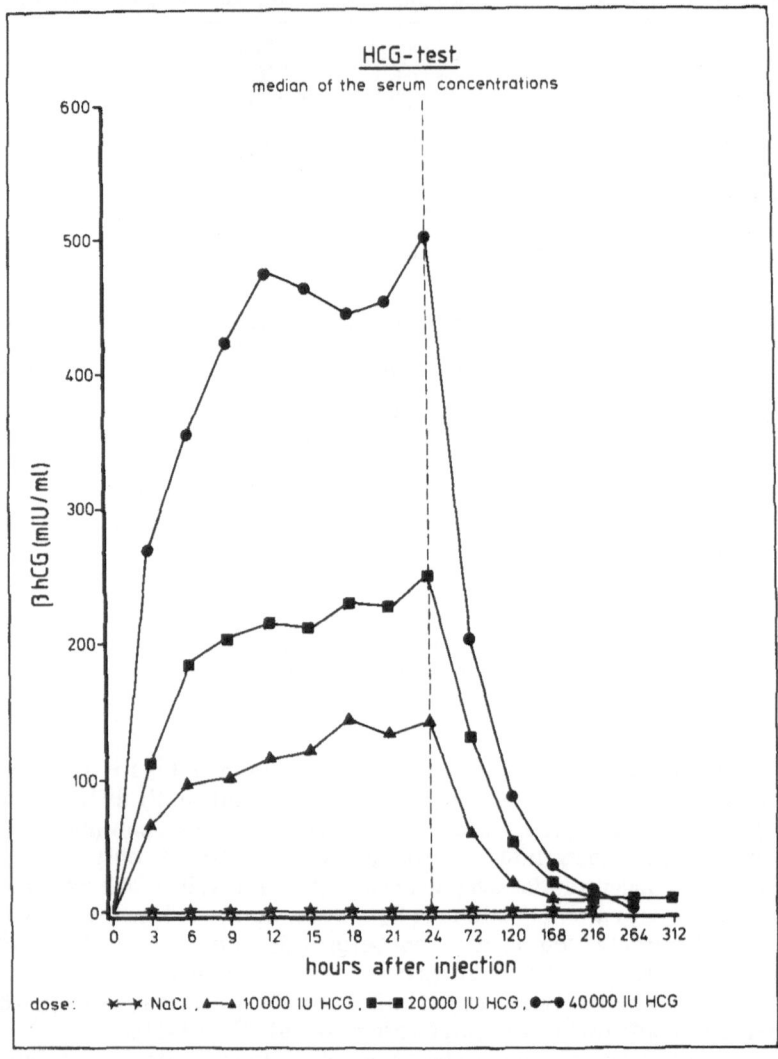

Figure 10.2 β-hCG serum concentrations (median) after injections of physiologic saline, 10 000, 20 000 and 40 000 IU hCG i.m. in 76 infertile women during the luteal phase

In the group of patients who had been administered saline, the concentrations of 17-OHP proved to have a significant circadian rhythm similar to the one in the corresponding P response curve (Figure 10.5). At all time intervals the hCG groups differed significantly from the placebo group. Only after 5 and 7 days did the various hCG dosages lead to significantly different results with 17-OHP reaching its lowest level after injection of 10 000 IU hCG and its highest concentration following injection of 40 000 IU hCG.

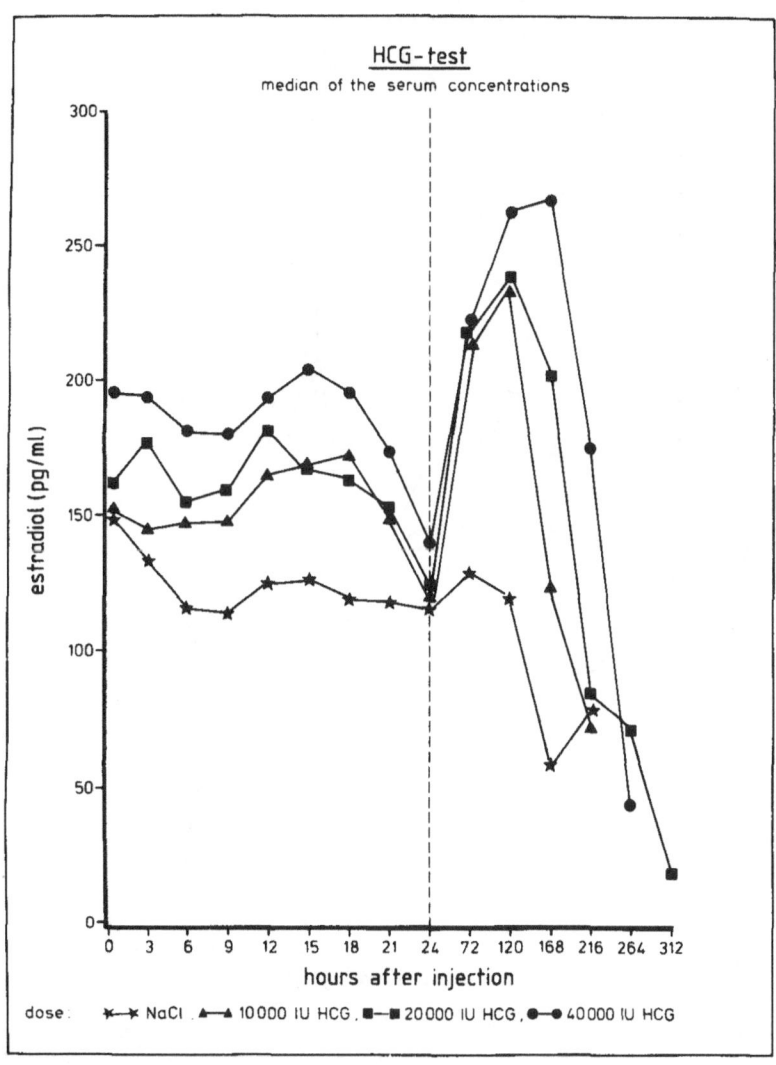

Figure 10.3 Estradiol-17β serum concentrations (median) after injections of physiologic saline, 10000, 20000 and 40000 IU hCG i.m. in 76 infertile women during the luteal phase

The prolactin response curves showed the already known significant circadian rhythm with higher values at night than during the day (Figure 10.6). No significant difference between the placebo group and the hCG groups could be demonstrated.

As hCG stimulation resulted in a higher secretion of all three steroids tested the question arose whether a possible interrelation of the steroids may be of importance. There was no relative difference between P and 17-OHP. The

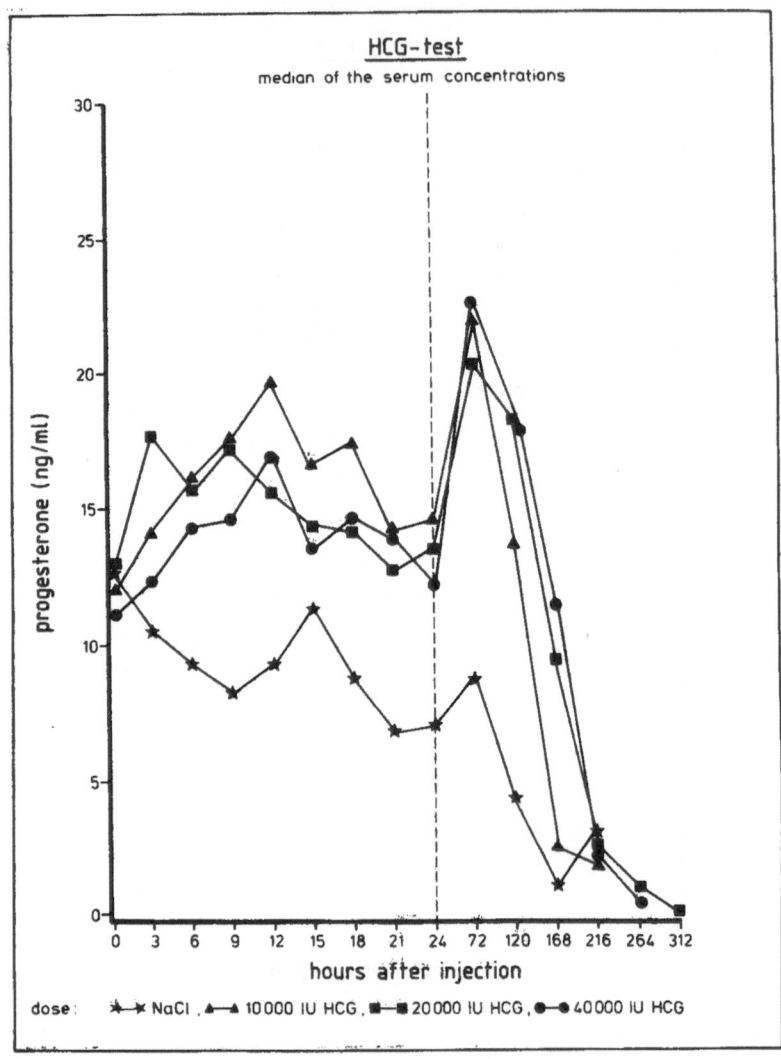

Figure 10.4 Progesterone serum concentrations (median) after injections of physiologic saline, 10 000, 20 000 and 40 000 IU hCG i.m. in 76 infertile women during the luteal phase

same applied for P and E_2, however, only until 18 h after administration of hCG. From 21 h up to the menstrual period the quantitative relation of P and E_2 changed significantly in favour of P. In the hCG group the 17-OHP/E_2 ratio was significantly higher 6, 9, and 24 h after injection. Of clinical importance was a significant dose-dependent prolongation of the luteal phase in all hCG test groups.

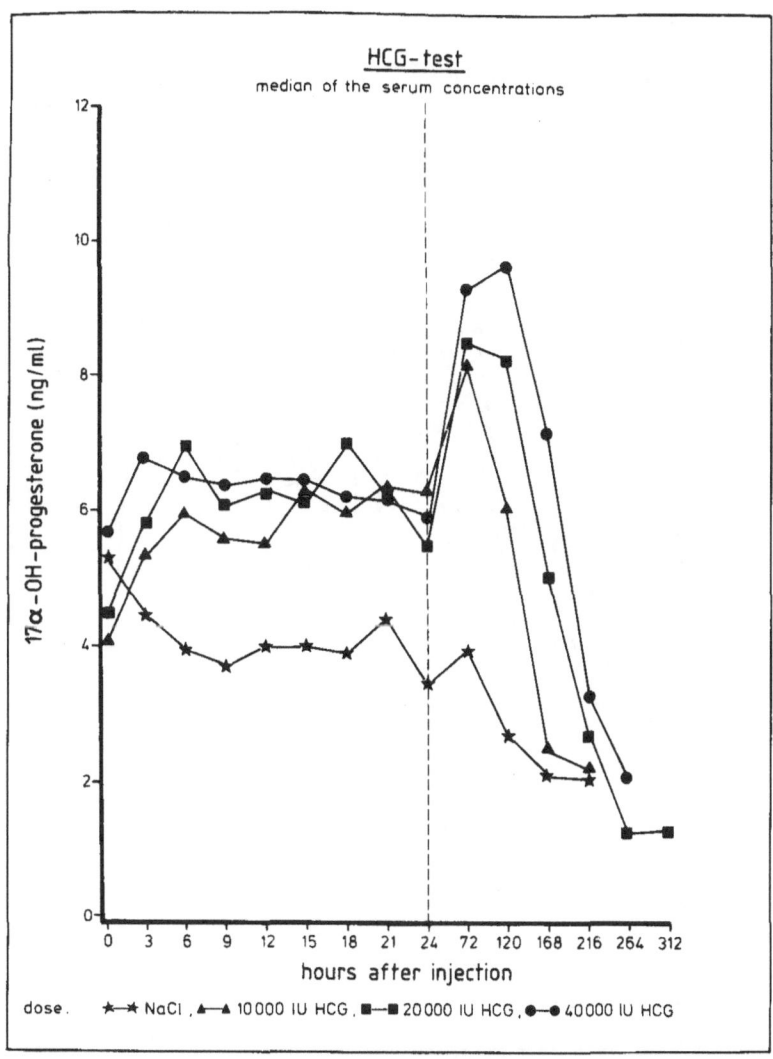

Figure 10.5 17α-hydroxyprogesterone serum concentrations (median) after injections of physiologic saline, 10 000, 20 000 and 40 000 IU hCG i.m. in 76 infertile women during the luteal phase

Before attempting an evaluation of the possible clinical importance of hCG-induced changes, several clinical items pointing to luteal insufficiency will be compared with the basal hormone value of all women and the hormone concentration charts of the placebo group.

The basal P concentrations showed a significant negative correlation with individual body weight ($r = -0.385$) and a significant positive correlation

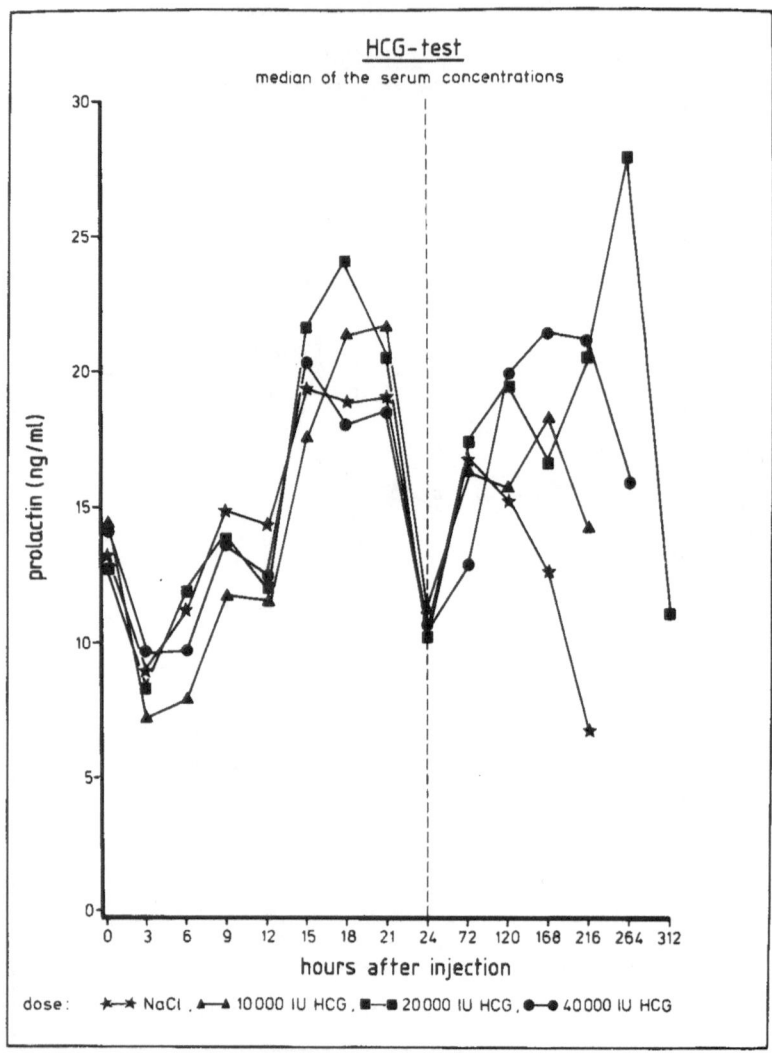

Figure 10.6 Prolactin serum concentrations (median) after injections of physiologic saline, 10 000, 20 000 and 40 000 IU hCG i.m. in 76 infertile women during the luteal phase

with 17-OHP concentrations ($r = 0.412$). The 17-OHP concentrations showed a positive correlation with the E_2 values ($r = 0.377$) and the P/E_2 ratio ($r = 0.685$). The prolactin concentrations were also positively correlated with the E_2 concentrations ($r = 0.345$) and showed a negative correlation with the P/E_2 ratio ($r = 0.658$). None of the clinical items had any interrelation with these basal hormone values.

A comparison of clinical data and the hormone concentration charts of the placebo group is given in Table 10.3. None of the chart characteristics showed

Table 10.3 Significant correlations between serial determinations of progesterone, 17α-hydroxyprogesterone, estradiol-17β, and prolactin and clinical items in the placebo group ($n = 19$). ($+$) positive correlation, ($-$) negative correlation, (0) no correlation

Items	Hormone	Characteristic of the "response" curve (24 h period)
1. Body weight	0	
2. Duration of infertility	Prolactin	($+$) Abs. val. 3 a.m.
3. Pregnancy after testing	0	
4. Day of ovulation	0	
5. Duration of luteal phase	Progesterone	($+$) Abs. val. 6–9 p.m.
		($+$) Integral net and percentage increase
	P/E_2	($+$) Abs. val. 6 p.m.–6 a.m.
		($+$) Min, max, integral
6. Progesterone basal value	Progesterone	($+$) Abs. val. 9 a.m.–9 p.m.
		($-$) Net increase 9 p.m.–9 a.m.
	17-OH-progesterone	($+$) Abs. val. 9 a.m.–3 p.m.

($+$), Positive correlation; ($-$), negative correlation; 0, no correlation. Abbreviations as Figure 10.1

a significant correlation with individual body weight or time of ovulation. The frequency of patients becoming pregnant was also independent of any hormone values. After prolonged infertility significantly higher prolactin concentrations were measured at night. Patients with a relatively short luteal phase appeared to have lower absolute P concentrations in the afternoon, and the integral of net and percentage increases was smaller. The P/E_2 ratio, as well as the minimum, maximum and integral values, were significantly smaller during the second half of the day and at night.

The dependence of the response curves on the basal P values was most pronounced. Low basal P values coincided with low P concentrations during the entire day. The net increase was, however, significantly higher at night. The basal 17-OHP concentrations showed a positive correlation with basal P values and in the case of low P values kept at a low level until the afternoon.

After hCG injection a number of interrelations of the hormone response curves with clinical data could be demonstrated (Table 10.4). At various time intervals after injection the body weight influenced the P concentration. In patients with a prolonged history of infertility a longer period of time elapsed until a maximum P concentration and P/E_2 ratio was reached. Women who became pregnant after testing showed a significantly higher P/E_2 and 17-OHP/E_2 ratio following 3 days after hCG injection. There was no correlation with the individual time of ovulation. The maximum of the P/E_2 ratio showed a significant correlation with the duration of the luteal phase. A positive correlation with the P/17-OHP ratio in the afternoon hours could also be demonstrated. In the afternoon and at night the 17-OHP/prolactin ratio was in inverse proportion to the length of the luteal phase.

A connection with basal P values could be established for the majority of changes in the P response curves (Table 10.4; Figure 10.7). To demonstrate this the medians of the P concentrations were plotted in two groups in

Table 10.4 Significant correlations between serial determinations of progesterone, 17α-hydroxyprogesterone, estradiol-17β, and prolactin and clinical items in women after hCG injections ($n = 57$)

Items	Hormone	Characteristics of the hCG-response curve
1. Body weight	Progesterone	$(-)$ Abs. val. 3 p.m., 6 a.m.
		$(-)$ Min. val.
		$(+)$ Percentage increase 3 a.m.
	P/17-OHP	$(-)$ Abs. val. 2 p.m., 3 a.m.
2. Duration of infertility	Progesterone	$(+)$ T max
	P/E$_2$	$(+)$ T max
3. Pregnancy after testing	P/E$_2$	$(+)$ Abs. val. 3 days
		$(+)$ T min
	17-OHP/E$_2$	$(+)$ Abs. val. 3 days
4. Day of ovulation	0	
5. Duration of luteal phase	P/E$_2$	$(+)$ Max
	P/17-OHP	$(+)$ Abs. val. 3–9 p.m.
	17-OHP/prolactin	$(-)$ Abs. val. 3 p.m.–3 a.m.
6. Progesterone basal value	Progesterone	$(+)$ All abs. values
		$(+)$ Min, max, T max, integral, integral net increase
		$(-)$ Net increase 9 a.m.–5 a.m. 7 days
		$(-)$ Percentage increase 9 p.m.– 7 days, integral percentage increase
	17-OHP	$(+)$ Abs. val. 9 a.m.–6 p.m.
		$(+)$ Min, max, integral
		$(-)$ Percentage increase 5 days

$(+)$, Positive correlation; $(-)$, negative correlation. Abbreviations as Figure 10.1

correlation with basal P values. All characteristics of the P response curves correlated with the basal P values, as well as with all ratios containing P. During the entire day the 17-OHP concentrations and the corresponding ratios also showed a positive correlation with basal P values.

After completion of the hCG test 26 out of 57 women became pregnant and 11 of them had abortions. In 20 patients non-ovarian sterility factors, none of them very marked, were found. However, the cause of sterility remained unclear in 11 cases. Examination of the hCG response curve in these four groups showed that the P/E$_2$ and 17-OHP/E$_2$ ratios 3 days after hCG application were highest in the group with later delivery and lowest in the case of unclear sterility. A sufficient corpus luteum function was assumed on the basis of a P/E$_2$ ratio of 0.12 and more. For another, the prolactin concentrations reached a night maximum in patients with abortion and in women with unclear cause of sterility.

When summarizing the hCG-induced hormone concentration changes, the basal P value proves to be of importance in so far as it obviously modulates the P and 17-OHP response curves. With regard to patients becoming pregnant following testing, the P/E$_2$ or 17-OHP/E$_2$ ratio 3 days after hCG injection could possibly be of clinical significance.

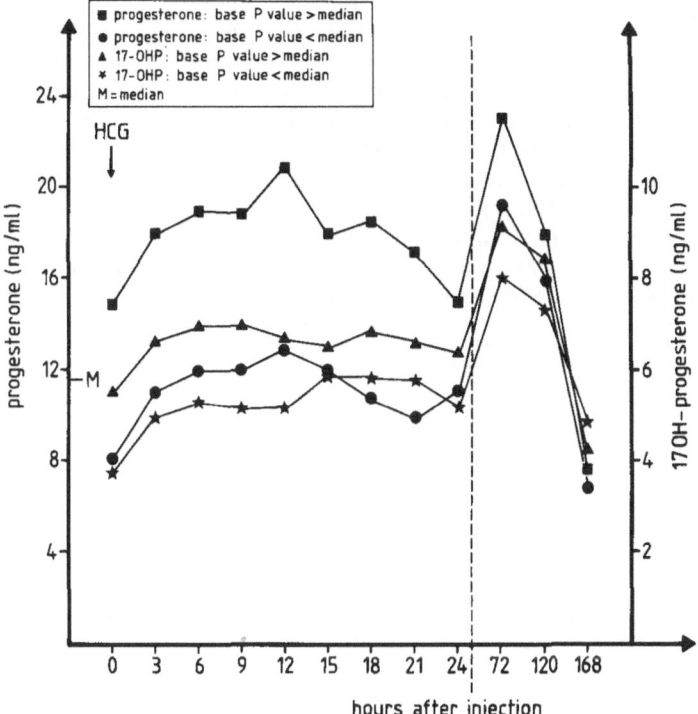

Figure 10.7 Serial progesterone and 17α-hydroxyprogesterone concentrations (median) in 57 women after i.m. injection of hCG. According to the basal progesterone values the patients were divided into those with basal P concentrations below the median (M) and those with basal P concentrations above the median

LH-RH TEST

The effects of various doses of LH-RH on the serum concentrations of FSH, LH and P were tested in 68 healthy women during the luteal phase of the menstrual cycle. Four groups of 13 women each received a single intra-muscular (i.m.) injection of 125, 250, 500 or 1000 μg LH-RH. After the injection blood samples were taken at 15 min intervals for 1 h, then at 60 min intervals for 8 h. In an additional 16 women the effect of two repeated injections of 1000 μg LH-RH given at different time intervals on day 5 of the luteal phase was examined. Blood samples were taken as described above and the concentrations of FSH, LH and P were radioimmunologically determined.

Mean LH levels increased sharply 15 min after the injection of LH-RH. There was a 10-fold increase of the LH concentration after 125 μg LH-RH and a 17-fold increase after 1000 μg. Peak concentrations were reached 1–3 h after injection. Up to 8 h after the injection of LH-RH, LH had not returned to its initial level.

In the case of FSH a similar pattern was found. Two hours after the injection of 125 μg LH-RH the mean FSH level increased 3-fold, and 3 h after 1000 μg LH-RH mean FSH concentrations reached a 6-fold peak. The peak was followed by a steep decline. For both gonadotropins a significant dose-dependent response was observed after injections of 125, 500 and 1000 μg LH-RH ($p < 0.01$). The response to 250 μg did not differ from that to 500 μg.

The mean P concentrations began to rise 45–60 min after the LH-RH injections (Figure 10.8). There was a 75–100% increase over mean baseline levels. The mean maximum levels were reached 3–7 h after the injection. Administration of 1000 μg LH-RH induced a biphasic pattern of elevation characterized by an early peak after 3 h and a late peak after 7 h ($p < 0.01$).

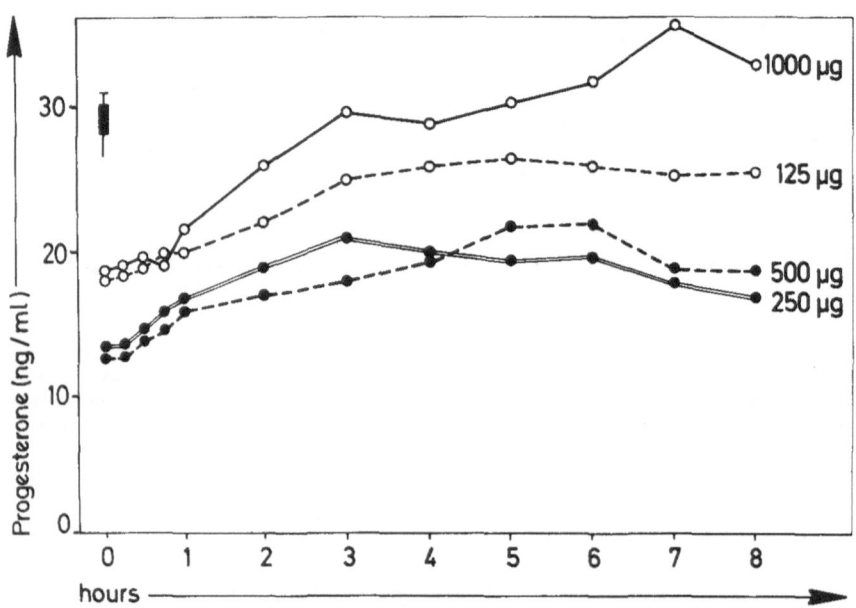

Figure 10.8   Mean serum levels of progesterone after i.m. injections of different LH-RH doses

The basal P values in the group of women tested with 250 and 500 μg LH-RH were significantly lower than the basal concentrations in the women receiving 125 and 1000 μg LH-RH. Comparable to the situation after hCG application the P secretion rate after LH-RH injection was dependent on the basal P concentrations. In the presence of identical basal concentrations a dose-dependence existed between 125 and 1000 μg LH-RH. The administered LH-RH dosages had obviously not been chosen in quantitative correspondence with the hCG injections. A comparison of the baseline levels of FSH and LH on the one hand, and P on the other hand, did not reveal any correlation.

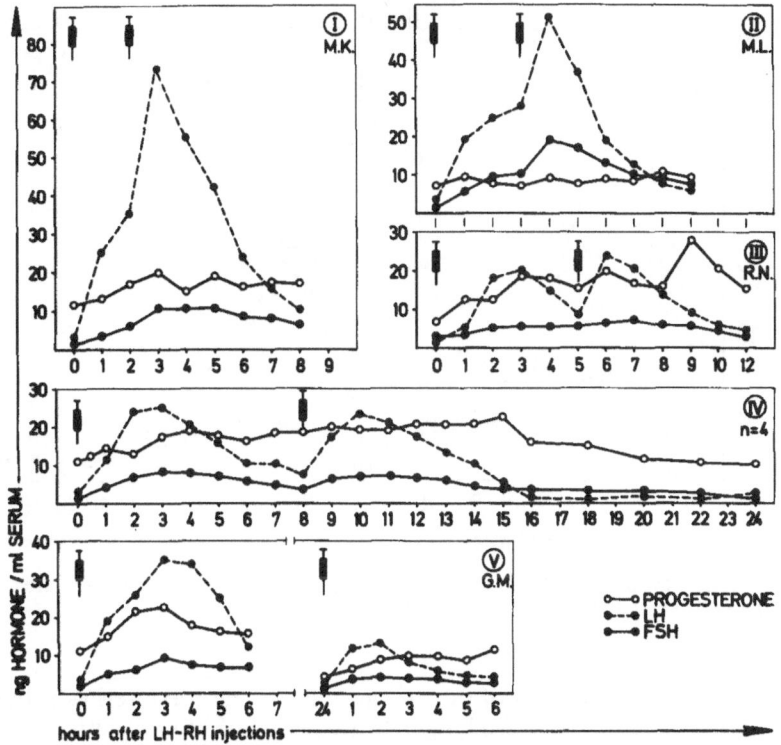

Figure 10.9 Serum levels of LH, FSH and progesterone after i.m. injections of 1000 μg LH-RH at different time intervals on day 5 of the hyperthermic phase. 1–2 h intervals, 2–3 h intervals, 3–5 h intervals, 4–8 h intervals, 5–24 h intervals

The repeated injections at 2 and 3 h intervals (Figure 10.9) induced cumulative effects on the increases of serum FSH and LH. When the second injection was given after 5 or 8 h, the LH and FSH response was within the same range as after the first stimulation. In these latter cases P concentrations which usually began to decrease after 8 h remained at a higher level for an additional 8 h. When the second injection was given 24 h later, a reduced response of FSH and LH was seen though the preinjection levels remained unchanged. P concentrations were significantly lower 1 day after the first injection. The second injection, however, resulted again in increased P concentrations.

Five women received 1000 μg LH-RH on days 5 and 7 of the hyperthermic phase. The mean values of FSH, LH and P are shown in Figure 10.10. The first stimulation showed a normal pattern with a 2-fold increase. After the second stimulation 48 h later the FSH and LH responses were significantly reduced. The mean basal P concentrations of day 7 were only half those of the 5th day. After the second injection the values increased 4.5-fold. The mean maximum P level was significantly lower after the second stimulation.

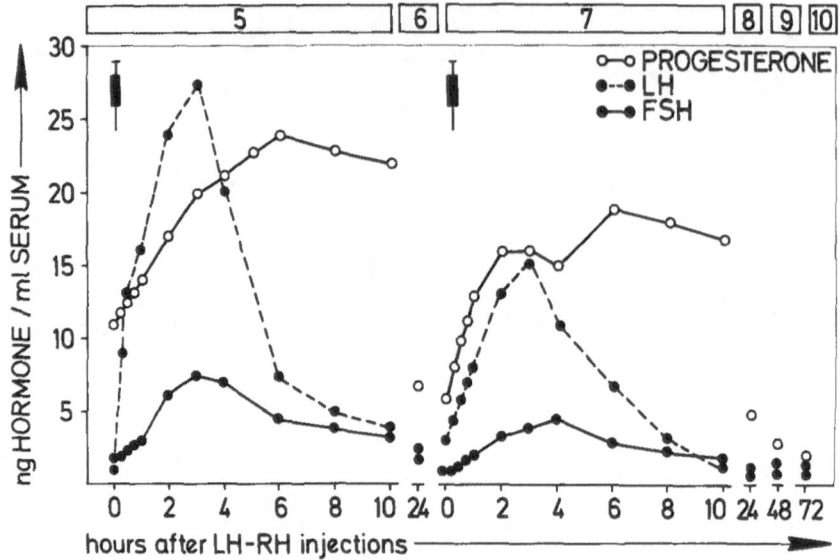

Figure 10.10 Mean serum levels of LH, FSH and progesterone in five women after i.m. injection of 1000 μg LH-RH on days 5 and 7 of the hyperthermic phase

Throughout the remainder of the treatment cycle, mean P levels were below the normal range. Due to the long half-life period of hCG the effect of this hormone on the corpus luteum is comparable to the situation after repeated brief-interval injections of LH-RH resulting in a prolonged stimulation of P. While the duration of the luteal phase was unchanged in women receiving a single injection of LH-RH or two repeated injections at less than 5 h intervals, the duration of the luteal phase was significantly reduced in the 10 women who were given repeated injections at more than 8 h intervals. We observed a mean of 13.6 days before the test and a mean of 9.6 days during the studied cycle ($p < 0.01$). Similar results were observed by Yen et al.[25] and Lemay et al.[21].

Considering these data an advantage of the LH-RH test over the hCG test for the evaluation of the corpus luteum function cannot be shown.

TRH AND METOCLOPRAMIDE TESTS

Within a prospective study, which has been carried out at our Department for one year, every patient is subjected to a detailed hormonal examination after clarification of tubal, andrological and immunological factors. So far the study comprises 74 women with biphasic cycles and normal basal concentrations of androgens, gonadotropins and prolactin. All patients showed a normal thyroid gland function in the TRH test.

136

In the early follicular phase (days 2–5 of the cycle) all basal hormone concentrations including prolactin were determined in blood pooled and drawn 3 times at 15 min intervals from an intravenous catheter. Fifteen and 30 min later, after an injection of 200 μg thyrotropin releasing hormone (TRH), blood was again drawn for determination of prolactin levels. During the luteal phase blood was collected three times between the 5th and 10th hyperthermic day for measuring P and E_2. Only the mean value of the three samples was considered for evaluation of the luteal phase. On one of the hyperthermic days a second blood sample was taken 30 min after injection of 10 mg metoclopramide. All serum hormones were radioimmunologically measured. The data were statistically analysed with the SAS program[26].

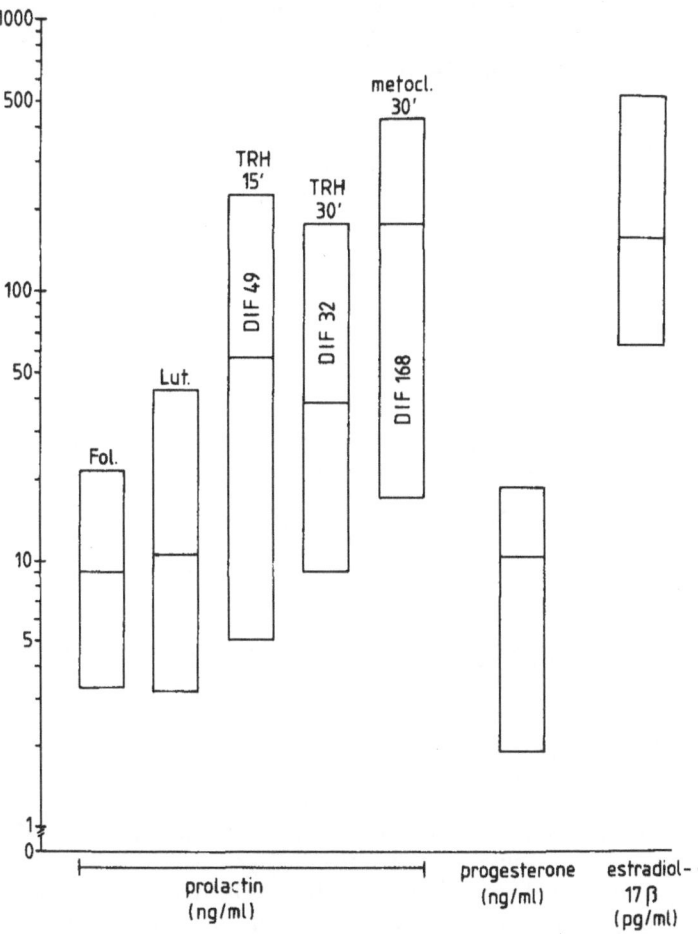

Figure 10.11　Serum concentrations of prolactin, progesterone and estradiol-17β in 74 women during early follicular phase (Fol, TRH) and luteal phase (Lut, metocl., progesterone, estradiol). Range of the values and medians are given. DIF = differences in ng/ml between prolactin levels after stimulation and basal prolactin concentrations

Figure 10.11 shows the serum concentrations of prolactin, P and E_2, with and without stimulation, in 74 women. Only the range and medians are given, as all hormones were spread according to standard logarithmic distribution. The differences between prolactin levels after stimulation and basal prolactin concentrations were also calculated.

The basal prolactin concentrations were significantly higher in the luteal phase than during the early follicular phase (Wilcoxon matched pairs test: $p < 0.002$). The difference between the basal value and the value following stimulation was 3–4 times higher after metoclopramide than it was after TRH.

A comparison of the hormone concentrations revealed no correlation between the concentrations of P, prolactin and E_2. A significant positive correlation with E_2 concentrations (Figure 10.12) could only be demonstrated for the prolactin levels 30 min after metoclopramide (Spearman correlation coefficient 0.3244; $p = 0.0229$).

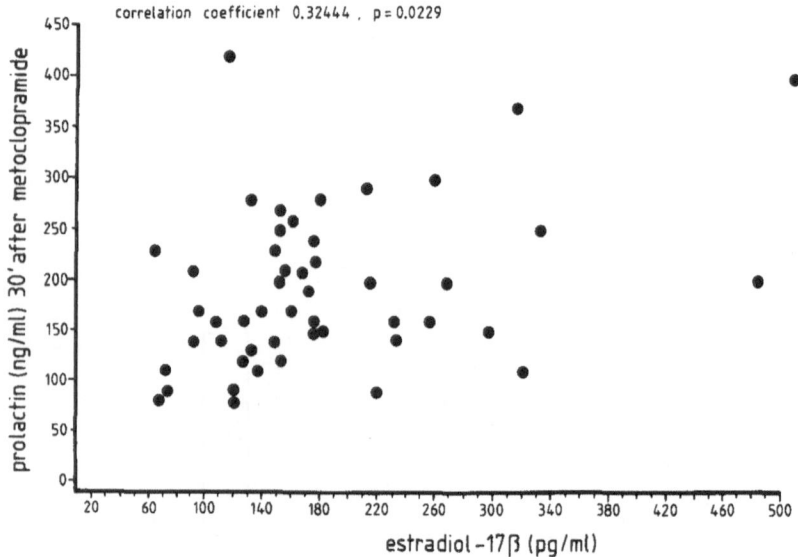

Figure 10.12 Correlation between the estradiol concentrations and prolactin concentrations 30 min after intravenous injection of metoclopramide during the luteal phase

In 15 women spontaneous gestation was observed during one of the following cycles. The Wilcoxon test was employed for ascertaining differing patterns of hormonal reaction (Table 10.5). All patients with spontaneous gestation had significantly reduced prolactin values during the follicular phase. During the luteal phase only the prolactin values after metoclopramide stimulation showed differences, while the concentrations of P and E_2 did not reveal any significant changes.

In addition to the above-mentioned 15 fertile women, seven patients

Table 10.5 Differences in the serum hormone concentrations between infertile women and women becoming pregnant after spontaneous ovulations in following cycles (Wilcoxon test)

Hormones	Median values (ng/ml)		Probability
	Pregnancy in following cycles (n = 15)	Infertile (n = 52)	
Prolactin fol.	7.2	10.0	0.01
Prolactin 15 min. TRH	40.0	58.0	0.02
Prolactin dif. 15 min. TRH	31.3	49.6	0.04
Prolactin 30 min. TRH	28.0	42.0	0.02
Prolactin dif. 30 min. TRH	20.3	32.9	0.05
Prolactin lut.	10.9	10.4	n.s.
Prolactin 30 min. metocl.	126.0	190.0	0.04
Prolactin dif. 30 min. metocl.	112.9	175.6	0.04
Progesterone	9.9	10.4	n.s.
Estradiol-17β (pg/ml)	151.0	157.0	n.s.

Abbreviations: fol. = follicle phase; lut. = luteal phase; 15 (30) min. TRH = minutes after intravenous injection of 200 μg thyrotropin releasing hormone; 30 min. metocl. = minutes after intravenous injection of 10 mg metoclopramide; dif. = difference between stimulated and basal values; n.s. = not significant

happened to conceive during the test cycle. While the hormone levels of the follicular phase were comparable in both groups, the luteal phase concentrations of P and prolactin after stimulation with metoclopramide were significantly higher in these early pregnant women ($p < 0.05$).

The preliminary results of these data stress the fact that though a correlation between the P and prolactin concentrations is missing, women with normal luteal function have significantly lower prolactin values in the follicular phase and after stimulation. The predictive value of the TRH test during the early follicular phase is comparable to that of the metoclopramide test during the luteal phase.

The following guidelines for the diagnostics of corpus luteum function are inferred from the results of hormone load tests on the basis of the studies conducted at our Department:

(1) Due to the circadian rhythms of the steroids examined, only the basal hormone concentrations at identical times of the day may be compared with each other.

(2) During luteal phase single determinations of P, 17-OHP, E$_2$ and prolactin with calculation of corresponding concentration ratios allow no reliable conclusions to be drawn with regard to the corpus luteum function.

(3) The prolactin levels in fertile women are significantly reduced during early follicular phase and at night during luteal phase.

(4) Every corpus luteum reacts to hCG or LH-RH stimulation with the secretion of P, the degree of which depends on the individual basal values. This implies that a purely ovarian cause of luteal insufficiency is obviously extremely rare.

139

(5)   The reactions of hCG and LH-RH are dose-dependent. Because of the different half-life periods of the two hormones LH-RH had to be reinjected at short intervals to obtain an effect comparable to that of hCG.

(6)   After hCG a double peak steroid response curve is observed for P, 17-OHP and E_2. Depending on the dosage the corpus luteum phase is prolonged. The prolactin concentrations remain unchanged.

(7)   The P/E_2 ratio 3 days after hCG is higher with fertile women than with infertile patients.

(8)   The relative excess of E_2 as demonstrated in the presence of the so-called luteal insufficiency leads to an intensified reaction of prolactin to TRH or metoclopramide stimulation.

References

1. Cooke, I. D., Morgan, C. A. and Parry, T. E. (1972). Correlation of endometrial biopsy and plasma progesterone levels in infertile women. *J. Obstet. Gynaecol. Br. Commonw.*, **79**, 647

2. Shephard, M. K. and Senturia, Y. D. (1977). Comparison of serum progesterone and endometrial biopsy for confirmation of ovulation and evaluation of luteal function. *Fertil. Steril.*, **28**, 541

3. Radwanska, E. and Swyer, G. J. M. (1974). Plasma progesterone estimation in infertile women and in women under treatment with clomiphene and chorionic gonadotropin. *J. Obstet. Gynaecol. Br. Commonw.*, **81**, 107

4. Abraham, G. E., Maroulis, G. B. and Marshall, J. R. (1974). Evaluation of ovulation and corpus luteum function using measurement of plasma progesterone. *Obstet. Gynecol.*, **44**, 522

5. Jones, G. S. (1976). The luteal phase defect. *Fertil. Steril.*, **27**, 351

6. Wentz, A. C. (1979). Physiologic and clinical considerations in luteal phase defects. *Clin. Obstet. Gynecol.*, **22**, 169

7. Wentz, A. C. (1980). Endometrial biopsy in the evaluation of infertility. *Fertil. Steril.*, **33**, 121

8. Andrews, W. C. (1979). Luteal phase defect. *Fertil. Steril.*, **32**, 501

9. Rosenberg, S. M., Luciano, A. A. and Riddick, D. H. (1980). The luteal phase defect: the relative frequency of, and encouraging response to, treatment with vaginal progesterone. *Fertil. Steril.*, **34**, 17

10. Rosenfeld, D. L., Chudow, S. and Bronson, R. A. (1980). Diagnosis of luteal phase inadequacy. *Obstet. Gynecol.*, **56**, 193

11. Downs, K. A. and Gibson, M. (1983). Clomiphene citrate therapy for luteal phase defect. *Fertil. Steril.*, **39**, 34

12. Sherman, B. M. and Korenman, S. G. (1974). Measurement of plasma LH, FSH, estradiol and progesterone in disorders of the human menstrual cycle: the short luteal phase. *J. Clin. Endocrinol. Metab.*, **38**, 89

13. Ross, G. T. and Hillier, S. G. (1978). Luteal maturation and luteal phase defect. *Clin. Obstet. Gynecol.*, **5**, 391

14. Perez, R. J., Plurad, A. V. and Palladino, V. S. (1981). The relationship of the corpus luteum and the endometrium in infertile patients. *Fertil. Steril.*, **35**, 423

15. Hull, M. G. R., Savage, P. E., Bromham, D. R., Ismail, A. A. A. and Morris, A. F. (1982). The value of a single serum progesterone measurement in the midluteal phase as a criterion of a potentially fertile cycle ("ovulation") derived from treated and untreated conception cycles. *Fertil. Steril.*, **37**, 355

16. Rice, B. F., Hammerstein, J. and Savard, K. (1964). Steroid hormone formation in the human ovary: II. Action of gonadotropins *in vitro* and in the corpus luteum. *J. Clin. Endocrinol.*, **24**, 606

17. Geiger, W., Kaiser, R. and Kneer, M. (1969). Herstellung von Pseudograviditäten bei Frauen durch hochdosierte der Frühgravidität angepaßte HCG-Gaben. *Acta Endocrinol., (Kbhv.)* **62**, 289

18. Hanson, F. W., Powell, J. E. and Stevens, V. C. (1971). Effects of HCG and human pituitary LH on steroid secretion and functional life of the human corpus luteum. *J. Clin. Endocrinol.*, **32**, 211

19. Runnebaum, B., Rieben, W., Bierwirth v. Münstermann, A.-M. and Zander, J. (1972). Circadian variations in plasma progesterone in the luteal phase of the menstrual cycle and during pregnancy. *Acta Endocrinol., (Kbhv.)* **69**, 731

20. Gerhard, I. and Runnebaum, B. (1982). The hCG test: an approach to luteal insufficiency. *Eur. J. Obstet. Gynecol. Reprod. Biol.*, **14**, 101

21. Lemay, A., Labrie, F., Ferland, L. and Raynaud, J. P. (1979). Possible luteolytic effects of luteinizing hormone-releasing hormone in normal women. *Fertil. Steril.*, **31**, 29

22. Bohnet, H. H., Hilland, U., Hanker, J. P. and Schneider, H. P. G. (1980). Epimestrol in der Behandlung der normoprolaktinämischen Corpus luteum-Insuffizienz. *Geburtsh. u. Frauenheilk.*, **40**, 926

23. Semple, C. G., Beastall, G. H., Teasdale, G. and Thomson, J. A. (1983). Hypothyroidism presenting with hyperprolactinaemia. *Br. Med. J.*, **286**, 1200

24. Goldstein, D., Zuckermann, H., Harpaz, S., Barkai, J., Geva, A., Gordon, S., Shalev, E. and Schwartz, M. (1982). Correlation between estradiol and progesterone in cycles with luteal phase deficiency. *Fertil. Steril.*, **37**, 348

25. Yen, S. S. C., Vandenberg, G., Rebar, R. and Ehara, Y. (1972). Variation of pituitary responsiveness to synthetic LRF during different phases of the menstrual cycle. *J. Clin. Endocrinol. Metab.*, **35**, 931

26. Helwig, J. T. and Council, K. A. (1979). *SAS Users Guide.* SAS Inst., Inc., Box 8000 Cary, NC 27511

Discussion

Taubert	How do you define a normal response in the metoclopramide test?
Gerhard	We consider the response as normal, if the injection of metoclopramide i.v. brings about an elevation of prolactin within 30 min to a value of not more than 200 ng/ml.
Insler	A short question, which you may not be willing or able to answer. After reviewing your data, would you like to suggest that one or possibly all these tests should be incorporated as a matter of routine into the diagnostic work-up of infertility?
Gerhard	I do think the TRH test should be done in any case, because you obtain both the response of prolactin and TSH. It should be performed in the early follicular phase. The metoclopramide test seems to provide similar information.
Bettendorf	What are the clinical consequences when you do this test?
Gerhard	The patients with an excessive response of prolactin to TRH will be treated with bromocriptine, and I will control the values of prolactin and progesterone during the luteal phase in order to reduce the dose, if necessary.
Peters	I do not think this is the right way to treat these patients. You should treat luteal dysfunction by other methods than bromocriptine, as it only reduces prolactin but does not normalize corpus luteum function.
Gerhard	I basically agree with your comment. We are at the moment conducting a prospective study in which the patients are treated in a randomized fashion with clomiphene, bromocriptine, or progesterone suppositories. When we consider our data, which comprise as yet not too many patients, there is so far no pregnancy on record. I do not know why everybody else seems to obtain such good results with progesterone suppositories. In contrast to women treated with the latter, we observed pregnancies both within the bromocriptine- and clomiphene-treated groups.
Dericks-Tan	I would like to know how pure is your hCG preparation as you measured β-hCG rather than hCG in serum? If you use a homogeneous β-hCG assay you are going to measure primarily β-hCG and its fragments. The cross-reaction with hCG is low, and β-hCG and its fragments have relatively low biological activity!
Gerhard	The hCG and β-hCG preparations were obtained from Serono, this will give you an idea of their purity. We are aware that we measure more or less only β-hCG. It would certainly be better to measure the whole hCG molecule, but we did not have that kind of assay at our disposal.
Rothchild	I have to take issue with you about the statement on the dose–response relationship between hCG, LH-RH, and progesterone, in spite of the good point you made that the responsitivity depends on the basal level.
Gerhard	In a previous study there was a significant dose-dependency at 5000 and 10000 IU. Higher doses in excess of 10000 IU hCG yielded identical results over a period of 24 h, but not at any time of the menstrual cycle. Due to the long half-life of hCG, the dose of 10000 IU brought about a prolongation of the luteal phase, and this was even more pronounced in the case of 40000 and 80000 IU, respectively.

DISCUSSION

Rothchild   Did all the patients suspected to have an inadequate corpus luteum respond equally well to hCG?

Gerhard   Yes, they all did respond.

Rothchild   This raises a question! I do not think that we know in what manner a population of normal women with a normal corpus luteum would respond to hCG. But if a corpus luteum suspected of being inadequate responds to hCG as well as a normal one does, why do we call it inadequate? How do we know that the patient bearing this corpus luteum would not have as much of a chance of becoming pregnant as a patient who had a normal corpus luteum? The eventual answer may come out in later papers, because the only way of being sure whether the corpus luteum is adequate or inadequate is, how it responds to treatment. And the only way to know whether the treatment has resulted in a response is to do a double-blind study.

Wentz   How did you make the diagnosis of luteal phase inadequacy in your patients, and secondly, was there an aetiologic breakdown of this patient population?

Gerhard   We started out with a group of infertile patients of as yet unknown cause. When the tests had been finished, we compared the duration of the luteal phase, the time of ovulation, and whether they had later become pregnant or not, etc. to the test results. That means we did not establish the diagnosis of luteal phase insufficiency before the tests, but classified the patients afterwards according to whether the progesterone values were above or below the median as having a sufficient or insufficient luteal phase.

Lehmann   Several years ago we also attempted to evaluate the function of the corpus luteum in patients suspected of suffering from luteal phase defect by means of a hCG-load test. The design of the test differed from yours, because it was conceived to accommodate patients who could not attend the infertility clinic for diagnostic purposes very often (Lehmann *et al.*, *Arch. Gynecol.*, **224** (1977), 424). We advised the patients to have an injection of 5000 IU hCG i.m. on the first day of menstruation, and to provide our laboratory with a blood sample drawn 3 days later. The injection brings about a reactivation of steroid synthesis in the regressing corpus luteum, and another increase in serum progesterone. We had made the observation that the progesterone values obtained 3 days after the injection of hCG reflect both in normal and in insufficient cycles the mid-luteal zenith of progesterone. The administration of 10 000 IU hCG gave even better results at the end of a normal luteal phase, but the reactivation of the corpus luteum function in insufficient cycles was found to be excessive. In the meantime we have discontinued the use of this test in favor of simpler diagnostic procedures such as the measurement of LH in morning-urine specimens by means of the HI-Gonavis or ultrasound examinations.

11
The luteinized unruptured follicle syndrome

P. R. KONINCKX and I. A. BROSENS

ABSTRACT

The existence of the luteinized unruptured follicle (LUF) syndrome has been firmly established. The data of the laparoscopic inspection of the ovaries have been confirmed by steroid hormone assays of peritoneal fluid and by the presence of the oocyte in the corpus luteum.

The LUF syndrome seems to be associated with endometriosis and it has been suggested that (mild) endometriosis might be the consequence of the LUF syndrome.

The role of the LUF syndrome as a cause of infertility remains unclear. The only evidence at present available is the finding that the syndrome occurs significantly more frequently in women with unexplained infertility than in a control group.

Diagnosis of the syndrome can be made by laparoscopic inspection of the ovaries, and by the assay of 17β-estradiol and progesterone in peritoneal fluid between day 14 and 20 of the cycle and probably by ultrasound.

The aetiology of the LUF syndrome is not yet known, but we favour the hypothesis that stress might be causally involved, since women with the LUF syndrome have a significantly higher trait anxiety than fertile women or infertile women without the LUF syndrome.

The treatment of the LUF syndrome is also unknown. Preliminary data suggest however that neither clomifene, nor gonadotropins, nor bromo-criptine are very effective.

INTRODUCTION

The idea of a luteinized, unruptured follicle (LUF) is not new. In the human, Stein and Leventhal suggested in 1935 rupture of the follicle beneath the cortex with entrapment of the oocyte and luteinization of the follicle. Similarly, 'ovulation', without release of the oocyte, was proposed to explain the discrepancy[1] between ovulation rate and pregnancy rate during clomiphene treatment. In the rat[2] and subsequently in the rabbit[3] and the monkey[4,5], it was demonstrated that a LUF syndrome can be induced by indomethacin treatment.

THE LUF SYNDROME EXISTS

Laparoscopic evidence

In 1978 two groups described independently that in women with infertility and apparently normal 'ovulatory' cycles, the ovulation ostium could often not be seen at laparoscopy[6–8]. This observation, however, does not prove that the LUF syndrome exists, since the ovulation ostium could have been re-epithelialized following ovulation, and since the ovulation ostium could have been missed or misinterpreted at laparoscopy.

The repair of the ovulation ostium has been studied in rats[9], rabbits and guinea pigs[10]. In these animals the ovulation ostium is covered by a layer of connective tissue cells within 2 days and re-epithelialized after 5–7 days. In the human the repair of an ovulation ostium has not yet been studied in detail. The animal experiments suggest, however, that an ovulation ostium will not be re-epithelialized before about a week following ovulation, and that it could thus be recognized as such during that period. In the human the repair process could even take a much longer time since the incidence of an ovulation ostium or scar in women with unexplained infertility, in women with pelvic endometriosis, and in a control group of women[6,7] was not significantly different between the early (days 14–20) and the late (days 21–28) luteal phase. Moreover, we occasionally observed an ovulation scar during the early follicular phase of the following cycle.

The accuracy of the laparoscopic inspection and the interpretation of an ovulation ostium has been subjected to much criticism. Unless ovarian mobility is limited, i.e. by adhesions, both sides of the ovary can always be inspected completely, either by using a dual puncturing technique, or by moving the uterus down and sidewards while the ovary is lifted out of the fossa ovarica. The evaluation of an ovulation ostium can be dubious (14%)[11], but in most cases the ostium can unequivocally be classified as absent (sometimes even a corpus luteum cannot be seen – sometimes the corpus luteum is cystic) or present. Even pictures can easily be recognized as such by everyone[11]. Final proof that this visual interpretation corresponded to some real phenomenon was given by the study of peritoneal fluid[11].

Biochemical evidence

In women with ovulatory cycles, according to their BBT, plasma progesterone concentrations and endometrial biopsies, the volume of peritoneal fluid increases progressively during the follicular phase, then abruptly at ovulation and declines progressively thereafter[12,13]. During the follicular phase concentrations of 17β-estradiol and progesterone[14] are slightly higher in peritoneal fluid than in plasma, but following ovulation the concentrations in peritoneal fluid increase sharply, and are some 5–10 times higher than in plasma. The differences between the free steroid hormone concentrations are still larger, since both transcortin and sex-hormone binding globulin concentrations are some 30% lower in peritoneal fluid than in plasma[14].

When this group of women with so-called ovulatory cycles was subdivided into women with and without ovulation ostium, we found that only women with an ovulation ostium have these very high concentrations of 17β-estradiol and progesterone in their peritoneal fluid following ovulation. Women without an ovulation ostium have barely elevated steroid hormone concentrations during the early luteal phase, except the women in whom the corpus luteum is cystic. These differences in 17β-estradiol or progesterone concentrations cannot be explained by differences in the concentrations of the binding proteins[11] nor by differences in the volume[13] of peritoneal fluid.

Peritoneal fluid data thus strongly support the concept of a LUF syndrome. Firstly, peritoneal fluid seems to be formed mainly by ovarian exudation[13]. Secondly, in order to maintain such a high concentration gradient of 17β-estradiol and progesterone between peritoneal fluid and plasma, up to day 20 of the cycle, continuous secretion of these steroid hormones into the peritoneal cavity has to be postulated. Thirdly, since steroid hormone concentrations are significantly higher when an ovulation ostium is present, we suggest that leakage of fluid through the ovulation ostium takes place. This fluid comes from the corpus luteum and is laden with estrogens and progesterone. When a luteinized unruptured follicle is formed, less exudation occurs with consequently lower steroid hormone concentrations in peritoneal fluid.

Ultrasonographic evidence

The ultrasonographic criteria of ovulation are well established. Using these criteria the frequent occurrence of a non-ruptured follicle which transforms into a corpus luteum, has been described[15]. However, at present no large-scale studies are available in which the ultrasonographic data are compared with laparoscopic inspection of the ovaries and with peritoneal fluid assays.

Presence of the oocyte in the corpus luteum

The final proof of a LUF syndrome, the presence of the oocyte in the corpus luteum, was recently demonstrated in the human as a case report[16]. For obvious reasons, studies of systematically enucleating the corpus luteum cannot be performed in women. In the rhesus monkey, however, it was demonstrated that in animals which developed a LUF syndrome following the induction of ovarian endometriosis, the oocyte was systematically present in the corpus luteum[17] (also R. S. Schenken, personal communication).

THE LUF SYNDROME IS A CAUSE OF INFERTILITY

The only available evidence, up to now, that a LUF syndrome is a cause of infertility, is the observation that the syndrome occurs statistically more frequently in women with unexplained infertility (incidence over 50%) than in a control group (incidence less than 10%).

Although there can be no doubt that a cycle with a LUF is infertile, repetition of the syndrome in successive cycles should be proven in order to accept it as a cause of infertility. This evidence is still not available since, for obvious reasons, laparoscopy cannot be performed in successive cycles. Ultrasonographic data, however, suggest repetition[18]. Moreover, one should be aware that repetition in each cycle is not absolutely required to induce infertility: a LUF syndrome still might reduce the probability of conception by reducing the number of fertile cycles.

ENDOMETRIOSIS IS ASSOCIATED WITH THE LUF SYNDROME

Endometriosis was found to be frequently associated with the LUF syndrome. Ovulation ostia were seen at laparoscopy in 94% of a control group of women, but only in 21% of patients with endometriosis and regular biphasic cycles. This difference was highly significant for mild, moderate and severe endometriosis[6]. This frequent occurrence of the LUF syndrome in women with endometriosis was subsequently confirmed by peritoneal fluid steroid hormone assays[19]. In the rhesus monkey it was, moreover, recently demonstrated that following the induction of ovarian endometriosis a LUF syndrome was almost systematically found[17].

Following the observation that viable endometrial cells in peritoneal fluid were present in almost 60% of women with or without endometriosis[19], the question arose as to why these endometrial cells did not implant more frequently. We suggest that this can be explained by the steroid hormone concentrations in peritoneal fluid, and the following hypothesis for the aetiology of endometriosis is proposed: endometrial cells, regurgitated during menstruation into the peritoneal cavity, are normally prevented from implanting on the peritoneum by the sex steroid hormone concentrations in peritoneal fluid. Whenever this inhibiting mechanism fails, as occurs when a LUF is formed, endometriosis may develop. Endometriosis thus would be the consequence, and not the cause, of infertility in such cases. Once established, however, and more particularly when the ovaries themselves are involved, endometriosis might aggravate infertility since ovarian function has been shown to be disturbed in women with moderate and severe ovarian endometriosis[6] and since ovum transport can be disturbed by tubo-ovarian adhesions.

RELATIONSHIP BETWEEN THE LUF SYNDROME AND 'SO-CALLED' LUTEAL PHASE INSUFFICIENCY

It should be clearly stated that all the women investigated in our studies had a luteal phase of normal duration. Women with a short luteal phase (11 days or less) were excluded.

In order to investigate the relationship of the so-called luteal phase insufficiency and the LUF syndrome we compared periovulatory plasma hormone concentrations and endometrial biopsy datings in women with regular cycles and a luteal phase of 12 days or more in women with and without a LUF syndrome. Plasma FSH concentrations in women with the LUF syndrome were significantly higher during 2 days following the LH peak than in women who ovulated. Contrary to this, preovulatory and peak concentrations were comparable in both groups of women. No clear-cut differences were found between the periovulatory concentrations of plasma LH, progesterone and 17β-estradiol, except that the 17β-estradiol peak occurred on the day before the LH peak in the ovulatory group but on the day of the LH peak in the women with the LUF syndrome. Prolactin concentrations, although slightly higher in women with the LUF syndrome, were comparable in both groups of women[20]. The duration of the luteal phase, defined as the interval between the LH peak and the onset of the next menstruation, was comparable in both groups of women: 13.4 ± 1.5 ($n = 12$) and 13.5 ± 1.2 ($n = 14$) days, respectively. Also, the dating of the endometrial biopsy was not different between the two groups of women. The delay between the expected day of the cycle as determined by the LH peak localization and the endometrial biopsy dating was 0.6 ± 1.7 days in the ovulatory group of women ($n = 8$) and 1.2 ± 1.1 days in the women with the LUF syndrome ($n = 12$)[20].

DIAGNOSIS OF THE LUF SYNDROME

Diagnosis of the LUF syndrome cannot be made by endometrial biopsy datings or plasma hormone assays. A LUF syndrome can, however, be suspected in those women in whom, after ovulation, the plasma FSH concentrations remain elevated for a few days.

Diagnosis can only be made by direct inspection of the ovaries, by ultrasonography and by peritoneal fluid assays of progesterone and 17β-estradiol. Between days 15 and 20 of the cycle, progesterone concentrations of more than 80 ng/ml and 17β-estradiol concentrations of more than 750 pg/ml were found, respectively, in 89% and 63% of peritoneal fluids in women with an ovulation ostium, whereas in women without an ovulation ostium these concentrations were found in only 25% and 20%. The use of both hormones together would lead to an accurate diagnosis of ovulation in 92% and 80% of women with and without an ovulation ostium, respectively[11]. The accuracy of the diagnosis by peritoneal fluid assays diminishes progressively as the luteal phase progresses, and disappears after day 19–20 of the cycle. The use of progesterone and 17β-estradiol concentrations in peritoneal fluid for the diagnosis of the LUF syndrome is further hampered by the fact that women with a cystic corpus luteum have high concentrations of both steroid hormones in their peritoneal fluid in spite of the absence of an ovulation ostium. A cystic corpus luteum probably constitutes such a large exudation area that the steroid hormone concentrations are elevated in spite of a LUF syndrome.

Since the evaluation of an ovulation ostium at laparoscopy may sometimes be difficult and eventually erroneous, the question should be asked if the diagnostic accuracy of peritoneal fluid assays is not higher than 92% and 80% in women with and without an ovulation ostium, respectively. The false positives and false negatives found could indeed be the consequence of ovulation ostia which were erroneously interpreted at laparoscopy.

AETIOLOGY OF THE LUF SYNDROME: A SPECULATIVE APPROACH

The mechanism which causes a LUF syndrome, is still unknown, but we speculated that the LUF syndrome might be caused by stress. When we assayed plasma prolactin concentrations in our women with infertility we were unable, however, to diagnose reliably moderate hyperprolactinaemia because of the frequent occurrence of stress hyperprolactinaemia[21]. Although we concluded that an infertility clinic is particularly stressful, the possibility that the patients are stress-prone cannot be excluded. Indeed, it is known that some subjects, i.e. neurotics, react to stress with a much more pronounced rise in prolactin and growth hormone concentration than a control group[22], while it is well known how 'stressed' women become when their infertility is not quickly solved. In order to evaluate this hypothesis women with the LUF syndrome, women with explained infertility and fertile women were evaluated by Spielberger's trait–state anxiety inventory (STAI) and it was found that women with a LUF syndrome have a significantly higher trait anxiety than both other groups of women[23]. We therefore suggest that the LUF syndrome might be causally related to stress. The LUF syndrome would thus become a mechanism for the 'so-called' psychological infertility[24, 25].

This hypothesis can furthermore explain many well-recognized but not yet understood facts in infertility, i.e. that 30% of all pregnancies of an infertility clinic occur during the investigations, the so-called spontaneous cure rate, even in women with long-standing infertility. The same phenomenon – an unexpected pregnancy – is seen relatively often in women with unexplained infertility, when therapy is stopped after years of treatment.

TREATMENT

Since the aetiology of the LUF syndrome is totally unknown, we do not yet know how to treat these patients.

Marik and Hulka[8] reported that 28 patients with unruptured luteinized follicles at the time of laparoscopy, and with no other obvious infertility factor, were treated with ovulation induction agents such as clomiphene and hMG. Fifteen of these patients subsequently conceived. Our results of the treatment of the LUF syndrome with ovulation stimulating agents or bromocriptine are certainly much lower (in preparation).

Since it is not yet proven that the LUF syndrome is constantly present in successive cycles, and since the LUF syndrome might explain the spontaneous cure rate in women with infertility, we want to stress that any form of treatment should be strictly assessed in comparison with a control group before conclusions are made.

Acknowledgements

We thank Professors M. Renaer, P. De Moor, and W. B. Robertson (St George's Hospital, London) and Professor G. Verhoeven, Dr W. Heyns, Dr W. Lissens, Dr H. Van Baelen, Professor Nijs and Dr Pijnenborg, co-authors of the articles reviewed. The assays were carried out predominantly by Mrs V. Celis and Mr B. Vanhalewijck. Mrs B. Minten and Mrs M. P. Vander Auwera are acknowledged for typing the manuscript.

References

1. Kase, N., Mroueh, H. and Olsen, L. E. (1967). Clomid therapy for anovulatory infertility. *Am. J. Obstet. Gynecol.*, **98**, 1037
2. Tsafriri, A., Lindner, H. R., Zor, U. and Lamprecht, S. A. (1972). Physiological role of prostaglandins in the induction of ovulation. *Prostaglandins*, **2**, 1
3. Armstrong, D. T., Grinwich, D. L., Moon, Y. S. and Zamecnik, J. (1974). Inhibition of ovulation in rabbits by intrafollicular injection of indomethacin and prostaglandin F2α antiserum. *Life Sci.*, **14**, 129
4. Wallach, E. E., De La Cruz, A., Hunt, J., Wright, K. H. and Stevens, V. C. (1976). The effect of indomethacin on HMG-HCG induced ovulation in the rhesus monkey. *Prostaglandins*, **11**, 727
5. Maia, H., Barbosa, I. and Coutinho, E. M. (1978). Inhibition of ovulation in marmoset monkeys by indomethacin. *Fertil. Steril.*, **29**, 565
6. Brosens, I. A., Koninckx, P. R. and Corveleyn, P. A. (1978). A study of plasma progesterone, oestradiol-17β, prolactin and LH levels, and of the luteal phase appearance of the ovaries in patients with endometriosis and infertility. *Br. J. Obstet. Gynecol.*, **85**, 246
7. Koninckx, P. R., Heyns, W., Corveleyn, P. A. and Brosens, I. A. (1978). Delayed onset of luteinization as a cause of infertility. *Fertil. Steril.*, **29**, 266
8. Marik, J. and Hulka, J. (1978). Luteinized unruptured follicle syndrome: a subtle cause of infertility. *Fertil. Steril.*, **29**, 270
9. Rosenbauer, K. A., Jansen, B. and Rapplund, S. (1976). Rasterelektronenmikroskopische Befunde an der Oberfläche des Rattenovars vor, während und nach der Ovulation. *Verh. Anat. Ges.*, 1053
10. Motta, P. and Van Blerkom, J. (1975). A scanning electron microscope study of the luteal follicular complex. II. Events leading to ovulation. *Am. J. Anat.*, **143**, 241
11. Koninckx, P. R., De Moor, P. and Brosens, I. A. (1980). Diagnosis of the luteinized unruptured follicle syndrome by steroid hormone assays on peritoneal fluid. *Br. J. Obstet. Gynaecol.*, **87**, 929
12. Maathuis, J. B., Van Look, P. F. A. and Michie, E. A. (1978). Changes in volume, total protein and ovarian steroid concentrations of peritoneal fluid throughout the human menstrual cycle. *J. Endocrinol.*, **76**, 123
13. Koninckx, P. R., Renaer, M. and Brosens, I. A. (1980). Origin of peritoneal fluid in women: an ovarian exudation product. *Br. J. Obstet. Gynaecol.*, **87**, 177
14. Koninckx, P. R., Heyns, W., Verhoeven, G., Van Baelen, H., Lissens, W. D., De Moor, P. and Brosens, I. A. (1980). Biochemical characterization of peritoneal fluid in women during the menstrual cycle. *J. Clin. Endocrinol.*, **51**, 1239
15. Coulam, C. B., Hill, L. M. and Breckle, R. T. (1982). Ultrasonic evidence for luteinization of unruptured preovulatory follicles. *Fertil. Steril.*, **37**, 524

16. Koninckx, P. R., Vasquez, G., Pynenborg, R. and Brosens, I. A. Presence of the oocyte in the corpus luteum of a woman with a LUF syndrome (submitted)
17. Schenken, R. S., Asch, R. H., Williams, R. F. and Hodgen, G. D. (1983). Etiology of infertility in monkeys with endometriosis. *Fertil. Steril.*, **39**, 393
18. Coulam, C. B. (1983). Ultrasonography and the LUF syndrome. *Fertil. Steril.*, **39**, 250
19. Koninckx, P. R., Ide, P., Vandenbroucke, W. and Brosens, I. A. (1980). New aspects of the pathophysiology of endometriosis and associated infertility. *J. Reprod. Med.*, **24**, 257
20. Koninckx, P. R., Brosens, I. A., Verhoeven, G. and De Moor, P. (1981). Plasma FSH levels in the luteinized unruptured follicle syndrome: a role for inhibin. *Br. J. Obstet. Gynaecol.*, **88**, 525
21. Koninckx, P. R. (1978). Stress hyperprolactinaemia in clinical practice. *Lancet*, **1**, 273
22. Miyabo, S., Asato, T. and Mizushima, N. (1976). Prolactin and growth hormone responses to psychological stress in normal and neurotic subjects. *J. Clin. Endocrinol.*, **44**, 947
23. Koninckx, P. R., Nijs, P., Verstraeten, D., Van Tendeloo, G. and Brosens, I. A. (1983). Increased trait anxiety in women with a LUF-syndrome (submitted)
24. Denber, H. C. B. (1978). Psychiatric aspects of infertility. *J. Reprod. Med.*, **20**, 23
25. Mai, F. M. (1978). The diagnosis and treatment of psychogenic infertility. *Infertility*, **1**, 109

Discussion

Rothchild	There are two points: (1) I agree that the absolute diagnosis is suggestive but somewhat subjective, and the only really good objective diagnosis would be the demonstration of the oocyte within the corpus luteum. Then, with the technique for ultrasonography which was described so beautifully in Chapter 8, by Dr Breckwoldt, I wonder why that would not just be the answer: here is a corpus luteum, and within it an oocyte. (2) I enjoy your speculations about the relationship between endometriosis, stress and prolactin. And while listening to the very interesting story, there did not seem to be much of a relationship, in fact, till I remembered some of the data that had been accumulating in our own laboratory about the relationship between prolactin and prostaglandins, and the importance of prostaglandins for the actual rupture of the follicle. Everybody should be reminded that prostaglandins are apparently absolutely essential for the follicle to rupture. Consequently, prostaglandins must be made within the follicle, and formation of prostaglandins is stimulated by the gonadotropins. Prolactin is important in inducing prostaglandin formation and function when its level is normal. Hyperprolactinaemic levels seem to inhibit the formation and function of prostaglandins.
Koninckx	What we are in fact lacking are data which combine the results of all diagnostic procedures, i.e. of ultrasonography, laparoscopy, and studies on peritoneal fluid. Secondly, I like your speculation on stress and prolactin. The change in skin-resistance as measured by a lie-detector occurs within seconds after exposure to stress. The reaction of prolactin differs from that. Moreover, the ovary is supplied by nerves just as the adrenal, the compensatory hypertrophy of which, e.g., has nothing to do with hormones, but is only brought about by a neural mechanism. There is some evidence that an ovarian disturbance may be mediated by a neural mechanism, too, the elevation of prolactin just being a side-effect.
Insler	I have a few technical questions. When did you perform laparoscopy to observe the stigma, and according to what parameters did you time the laparoscopy? How did you obtain the peritoneal fluid, in all cases by laparoscopy or by puncture of the space of Douglas? You showed, in your illustrations, differences in the concentration of different materials in the peritoneal fluid along the menstrual cycle; was this done on different women or were there repeated punctures on the same women?
Koninckx	All the peritoneal fluid samples were taken by aspiration through the laparoscope. We only had one sample in one woman under general anaesthesia. The prolactin concentration in plasma is very high under general anaesthesia, 2000–4000 μg/ml. The prolactin concentration in the peritoneal fluid is very high, too, about 2000 μg/ml. This may be normal because of the high plasma concentration even though it surprised us to see prolactin entering the peritoneal fluid from plasma so rapidly.
L'Hermite	I wonder with respect to the role of prostaglandins in follicular rupture whether anyone has been investigating women taking chronically drugs known to alter prostaglandin metabolism, e.g. aspirin. It would be

153

interesting to follow them with echography. I may have missed it, but have you correlated in your study concerning state- and trait-anxiety and in the same patients the effective prolactin levels to the results of the tests? It is easy to say that they are stressed, and prolactin is up. And what does stress mean? In animals we know that acute stress will increase prolactin but continuous stress will lead to depletion of prolactin and gonadotropin secretion.

Koninckx To answer the last question about stress and prolactin: we measured prolactin in the clinic, and obtained data which did not show any obvious difference.

Schweppe We found with sonography in patients with endometriosis proven by laparoscopy and biopsy in 12 cases out of 40 patients a LUF; but we also found in 10 cases out of 40 infertile patients, in whom endometriosis was excluded as a cause of infertility by laparoscopy, a LUF. That is, in our infertile patients the incidence is quite high, but there is no difference with regard to endometriosis.

The very interesting hypothesis of the induction of endometriosis by LUF is something like a vicious circle: you never can tell what comes first.

Koninckx That is why I was avoiding talking about the incidence of the LUF syndrome in different groups. I think it depends somewhat on where you are working. The incidence will be higher if you are working with patients who have been treated for infertility for some time.

Schneider Dr Rothchild mentioned the importance of the prostaglandins for follicular rupture. It has been demonstrated in rabbits that treatment with indomethacin or aspirin prevents follicular rupture. If you then inject PGE_2 into the follicle, they will rupture. So I wonder why you think that a neural mechanism has to be involved in the phenomenon of non-rupturing follicles?

Lehmann We know that the catecholamines are a certain factor in the accumulation process of the prostaglandins in the major follicles. If there is a stress situation, a disbalance between $PGF_{2\alpha}$ and PGE_2 may develop, or there is no accumulation of PGE_2 in the follicle. This may prevent ovulation.

Koninckx The prostaglandins fit definitely into this picture. It was also demonstrated in the rhesus monkey that indomethacin can induce a LUF syndrome.

Rothchild I think it is necessary to remind everybody here involved in the treatment of patients with infertility, that there is a tremendous psychosomatic aspect. I think, what Dr Koninckx is saying is that here is perhaps one mechanism through which the emotional disturbances may be responsible for infertility.

Dericks-Tan We have measured the proteo-hormone concentrations and the steroid concentrations in peritoneal fluid samples of about 70 patients and seldom found prolactin concentrations exceeding $500\,\mu IU/ml$ in the peritoneal fluid, even though in serum it was very high.

Bettendorf That would be in contrast to that what Dr.Koninckx said.

Koninckx Perhaps it was a difference in anaesthesia. In our patients the level was about $2000\,\mu IU/ml$.

Runnebaum In the resistant-ovary syndrome the maturation of the follicle is disturbed. Does the LUF syndrome occur in these patients too? Are there any indications for the development of a LUF syndrome in polycystic ovary syndrome?

Koninckx I always have problems with the definition of polycystic ovary. About 20% of women with polycystic ovary syndrome are in fact ovulating, and I would rather not answer that question because of the lack of definition.

Lehmann There is the question of how to treat these women which you excluded very nicely in your presentation. Do you try at first to exclude endometriosis in these patients, or do you first consider cyclic therapy? How many pregnancies, if any, have you seen after the therapy?

154

DISCUSSION

Koninckx   At this moment there are very beautiful data coming up about endometriosis. The management of minimal endometriosis with or without treatment gave about the same incidence of pregnancies in a double-blind prospective study. We have the impression that we are faced with approximately the same situation with the LUF syndrome. Because we thought it was an anovulatory condition, the patients were treated with clomiphene as an initial treatment, and we obtained about 40% pregnancies after 8 months of treatment. This incidence is exactly the same incidence which we have seen in women treated with clomiphene for anovulatory infertility.

Insler   Mr Chairman, if stress is the reason for the LUF-syndrome, the treatment would be love! Could we not agree to that.

Breckwoldt comments in writing as follows:

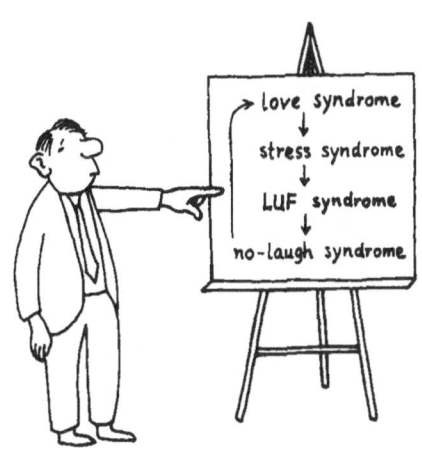

Section 3
Treatment

12

Progesterone supplementation for treatment of luteal phase inadequacy

A. C. WENTZ

INTRODUCTION

Progesterone supplementation for treatment of luteal phase inadequacy has received little critical attention. Although its use is widely recommended, there are few descriptions of the therapeutic approach and essentially no documentation of efficacy. Jones and Pourmand[1] reported an 80% pregnancy rate in 15 patients with primary infertility treated with intramuscular progesterone substitution therapy. Soules and co-workers[2] reported 16 infertility patients diagnosed to have luteal phase deficiency who were treated with progesterone supplementation by vaginal suppositories, with a 50% pregnancy rate. Katayama et al.[3], using a computer analysis in patients with primary infertility, found a cumulative 60% pregnancy rate in 33 cases of luteal phase inadequacy. Rosenberg et al.[4] diagnosed luteal phase inadequacy in 32 of 396 infertile patients (8.1%); 9 of 13 whose infertility was not complicated by other abnormalities conceived on progesterone supplementation and 7 of 13 carried to term. Balasch et al.[5] compared progesterone vaginal suppositories with dehydrogesterone in 44 infertile patients with an inadequate luteal phase, and documented a 62.5% pregnancy rate in 16 patients treated with progesterone; four patients delivered at term and one miscarried. In most of these series there was no consistent approach to the diagnosis, and criteria were not prospectively established as to choice of therapy where other modalities were available. Results of progesterone treatment are therefore difficult to interpret, and the efficacy and appropriateness of its use have been questioned. We have recently reviewed our patient population to address these points, and have concluded that progesterone supplementation is an appropriate first approach to therapy in selected patients diagnosed to have luteal phase inadequacy.

BACKGROUND

Pathophysiology of luteal inadequacy

The dependence of normal luteal hormonal output on preovulatory follicular development is now accepted[6-8]. Progesterone secretion is the primary function of the corpus luteum and is required for normal implantation and placentation. An adequate progesterone production ensures the ordered histological progress from a proliferative to a secretory endometrium, and the pattern of endometrial development reflects the adequacy of progesterone output as well as the ratio of progesterone-to-estradiol throughout the luteal phase. The correlation of endometrial dating with the onset of menses provides a bioassay of progesterone output; only measurement of serial peripheral progesterone concentrations provides comparable information[9]. The report by Keller and colleagues[10] describing a patient with persistent infertility, an inadequate endometrial response in the presence of normal progesterone output, and a proposed progesterone receptor defect at the level of the endometrium, stresses the importance of endometrial development for implantation and the necessity to evaluate the endometrium directly.

Jones, in 1949, described two forms of luteal phase inadequacy – the first due to a deficiency of progesterone output, and the second due to a defective endometrial response to hormonal stimulation[11]. The recent tendency has been to focus on the first, as shown by the numerous reports attempting to document luteal phase adequacy in terms of luteal hormone secretion and ratios[12-16]. However, several clinical situations have been described in which the endometrium has shown a defective response in face of an entirely normal progesterone output. For this reason we have preferred to define luteal phase inadequacy in terms of the endometrial pattern.

No signs or symptoms suggest the presence of luteal phase inadequacy due to a progesterone deficiency or to an inadequate endometrial response[17-33]. The basal temperature chart provides no quantitative information, and only an imprecise suggestion of luteal phase length. No characteristic change in menstruation, either in amount or duration of flow, correlates with the diagnosis. Recognizing the presence of luteal phase inadequacy is impossible without a definitive diagnostic test. If the endometrial biopsy is routinely included as part of the initial diagnostic approach to the infertile patient, then neither type of luteal phase inadequacy will be missed in the routine infertility evaluation.

Luteal phase inadequacy with no apparent derangement of follicular maturation or luteal function, and with normal progesterone levels, may be diagnosed by the identification of an inadequately prepared endometrial target organ. For example, a deranged endometrial pattern has been reported in patients resuming cyclic menstruation after discontinuation of danazol, with a septate uterus, with a proposed progesterone receptor defect, with Asherman's syndrome, with acute and chronic endometritis, and with submucous myomata[34-36].

Diagnosis of luteal inadequacy

The endometrial biopsy therefore has been used both as a bioassay of progesterone and estradiol output and as a means to assess normality of the implantation site. We have felt that consistency in the technique of biopsy, in its interpretation, and in the choice of therapy are essential. The biopsy must be taken from the fundus, and should represent a full thickness of the endometrium; lower uterine segment endometrium does not respond as completely to hormonal stimulation and an intact surface epithelium; the capsule is needed for accurate dating after ideal day 23 of the 28-day cycle. The late luteal phase biopsy reflects the stimulation from the entire span of luteal function, and the capability of the endometrium to respond appropriately to estrogen and progesterone. The endometrial biopsy taken on ideal day 26 or 27 is also the easiest to read histologically. The biopsy is assigned a date encompassing a 48-h span (e.g. secretory day 25–26), and the clinician needs to know only the date the biopsy was taken, the date of subsequent menstruation, and the histological reading of the biopsy to diagnose normality or a lag, the so-called out-of-phase biopsy. Because the endometrial pattern prior to menstruation should be similar, menses is chosen as the reference point, and arbitrarily called day 28. A biopsy obtained, for example, 2 days before menses should histologically appear as day 26; a pattern compatible with secretory day 22 would be abnormal. To make the diagnosis of an inadequate luteal phase, the biopsy must be out-of-phase, or lag the expected pattern by 2 days or more, and this finding should be verified in another menstrual cycle.

Obtaining the endometrial biopsy at the time of anticipated implantation, approximately day 21–22 of the ideal cycle, is not recommended. This endometrium is difficult to date, easily confused with an earlier pattern, and reflects only 7 days of progesterone exposure.

Taking the biopsy with the onset of menses has been recommended to avoid interrupting a pregnancy. However, once menstrual breakdown has begun, the integrity of the capsule and its underlying areas are destroyed, the degree and intensity of the generalized pseudodecidual response cannot be evaluated, and the biopsy cannot be accurately dated. Further, endometrial biopsy in the cycle of conception is apparently benign[37, 38].

Other approaches to diagnosis have not provided the same convenience and reproducibility. The ready availability of accurate serum progesterone measurements has made a blood test an attractive alternative, but serum progesterone levels will not reflect endometrial adequacy. Single or several mid-luteal progesterone levels have been used as an indicator of luteal phase inadequacy; Rosenberg[39] discussed the inappropriateness of using a single mid-luteal progesterone level for diagnosis. Rosenfeld and Garcia[40] reported a poor correlation between biopsy and progesterone results and made the important observation that if progesterone levels alone had been used for diagnosis, endometrial inadequacy would have been missed in 21% of their patients who had progesterone levels greater than 15 ng/ml. Balasch et al.[41] examined the usefulness of three samples, pooled as suggested by Abraham et al.[42], and found that 21.5% had an abnormal endometrial pattern in the face of normal progesterone output using Abraham's criteria. Accordingly, we have consistently used the endometrial biopsy in preference to serum progesterone measurements as the most direct means of assessing normality of the implantation site.

Treatment of luteal inadequacy

Treatment of luteal phase inadequacy begins with an investigation to determine the aetiological factor causing the inadequacy. The therapeutic approach to luteal phase inadequacy depends upon identifying specific causes and correcting the hormone deficiency involved. Every effort should be made to correct the primary cause of the condition.

Hyperprolactinaemia has been documented to be associated with luteal phase inadequacy; therefore the prolactin level must always be measured when luteal phase inadequacy is identified. Since hyperprolactinaemia can be associated with hypothyroidism, thyroid stimulating hormone (TSH) must be measured since treatment of existing hypothyroidism may result in normalizing the prolactin level.

Patients with a long follicular phase are manifesting derangements of folliculogenesis, and may have resultant luteal phase inadequacy. Aksel[43] and Broom and co-workers[44] have documented that cycles with ovulation intervals of 34–40 days ordinarily have normal luteal phase hormonal activity and endometrial response; in patients with a longer interval, clomiphene stimulation, and not progesterone supplementation, would be the treatment of choice.

Certain drugs, for example progestational agents and estrogens, can be luteolytic[45] and/or induce an endometrial glandular–stromal disparity. Estrogen vaginal creams, perhaps prescribed for cervical mucus problems, may inadvertently be used in the luteal phase as a coital lubricant.

A deranged endometrial pattern is seen with submucous myomata, an acute and chronic endometritis, and the septate uterus, so these too should be considered in the differential diagnosis.

Patients who are runners, or excessively thin, can be counselled as to the reproductive implications, although frequently these individuals are resistant to changing life habits. Perimenopausal patients probably require ovulation stimulation and not progesterone supplementation, particularly if cycle length is prolonged; a short luteal phase may respond to substitutional therapy.

There are several approaches to correcting the endometrial inadequacy. Progesterone administration is the most logical approach to treating what is probably a progesterone deficiency, either of output or response. Progesterone supplementation or replacement by vaginal or rectal self-administration has been our primary mode of therapy and has proved to be simple, effective, uncomplicated, and relatively inexpensive. Alternatively, luteal function may be stimulated, either directly using a luteotropic agent, or indirectly by stimulation of folliculogenesis.

Progesterone substitution therapy

Once the diagnosis of luteal inadequacy is clearly established according to the criteria of two biopsies, at least 2 days out-of-phase in two cycles, and other treatable aetiologies have been ruled out, then progesterone supplementation can be begun. The suppository can be manufactured inexpensively using the following simple formula to make 440 suppositories each 25 mg.

Progesterone powder	11 g
Polyethylene glycol 400	524 g
Polyethylene glycol 6000	348 g

To prove that the endometrial defect has been corrected, a repeat biopsy must be obtained in a treatment cycle. Too early administration of progesterone can inhibit ovulation, so some care must be taken as to when to begin the suppositories.

For most women, an elevated temperature, usually 97.8 °F (36.5 °C), reflects that presumptive ovulation has occurred. The progesterone suppositories are started when the temperature has been at or above this point for at least three consecutive days; therapy is never started before day 14 of the cycle. The vaginal suppository is inserted twice daily at 12 h intervals, and continued until the onset of the next menses, which is rarely delayed more than 2 days. The patient should be assured that the progesterone is rapidly absorbed, and that the expected vaginal leakage does not contain the active ingredient.

If the follow-up biopsy indicates that the endometrial defect has not been corrected, the simplest approach is to try suppository administration every 8 h. Alternatively, progesterone-in-oil 12.5 mg daily, self-injected, may be effective. If the endometrial defect has still not been corrected, some local problem, a submucous myoma, polyp or even a receptor defect, should be considered after checking plasma progesterone, which will be 10–15 ng/ml some 2–4 h after administration[46].

Progesterone levels achieved with replacement suppository therapy do not exceed those expected in the normal luteal phase and an appropriate pseudo-decidual and glandular response is observed. Progesterone has been found to be the most efficient drug in this respect; synthetic progestational agents produce unusual endometrial responses, particularly a developmental disparity between glands and stroma in which the glands are inadequately developed and the stroma maximally pseudodecidualized[47,48].

CLINICAL METHODOLOGY

All infertility patients, and those presenting with recurrent miscarriage routinely, were biopsied late in the luteal phase, as close to expected menses as possible. The endometrial biopsy was dated by the criteria of Noyes et al.[49], and correlated with the onset of next menses. For the diagnosis of luteal phase inadequacy to be established, two biopsies must be greater than 2 days out-of-phase in two menstrual cycles. An exception to the two-biopsy rule was made with patients presenting with recurrent miscarriages who were treated in the subsequent cycle and those taking clomiphene for ovulation induction, in whom a dosage change was made for the next cycle.

If luteal phase inadequacy was diagnosed by biopsy criteria, the attempt was made to determine the aetiology. Patients with a long follicular phase, hyperprolactinaemia, hypothyroidism, low body weight, and those at the extremes of reproductive life, were not candidates for progesterone supplementation as the treatment of choice. Those with a long follicular phase were started on clomiphene therapy, with the understanding that induction of ovulation using clomiphene could be expected to result in luteal phase inadequacy in perhaps 30–50% of treated patients[22, 23]; adequate luteal function was assessed in the first ovulatory cycle, and if an abnormality was found the clomiphene dose was usually adjusted upward. For patients undergoing ovulation induction as treatment for a more serious disorder of folliculogenesis, the approach was identical: biopsy in the first treatment cycle, and with diagnosis of luteal inadequacy, an increase in clomiphene dose to see if increased FSH stimulation might correct the problem; if not, then progesterone supplementation was added. Patients with hypothyroidism, hyperprolactinaemia and nutritional problems were managed with appropriate medical therapy. Patients at the extremes of reproductive life, particularly those over age 35, were treated with clomiphene, because of the supposition that they have abnormalities of folliculogenesis, rather than problems with endometrial response.

When these diagnostic groups were eliminated, there remained a number of women in whom no aetiology was discovered to explain the luteal phase inadequacy. In these patients progesterone supplementation was used as the initial treatment.

RESULTS

We identified 79 women with suspected luteal phase inadequacy evaluated as described above. The first endometrial biopsy was out-of-phase in 70 of these women presenting with infertility or early pregnancy wastage. In nine women considered to be at risk for luteal phase inadequacy, the first biopsy was equivocal, taken too early or out-of-phase by a single day on ideal day 25 (Table 12.1). These nine underwent another biopsy, which was out-of-phase in eight women; the remaining woman was biopsied in the cycle of conception (COC), and went on to deliver uneventfully.

Fifty-three of the 79 women had a second biopsy, which was out-of-phase in 45 (85%), in-phase in five (9%), and taken in the cycle of conception in three women, all of whom delivered. The five whose second biopsy was in phase deserve mention because three of the five had biopsies taken too early, before ideal day 25 of the cycle. Twenty-six of the initial 79 women did not undergo a second endometrial biopsy. In seven women, progesterone supplementation was added when clomiphene-induced inadequacy was diagnosed.

Table 12.1 Results of first and second endometrial biopsies

Biopsy 1		Biopsy 2				
In phase (IP) (n)	Out of phase (OOP) (n)	n	IP	OOP	COC*	No Bx
9		9	0	8	1	0
	70	44	5†	37	2	26
		53	5	45	3	26

*COC = cycle of conception
†Four taken too early, before ideal day 25
IP = in phase; OOP = out of phase; Bx = biopsy

Overall, for the entire series, including those who fulfilled strict criteria and those who did not, 61 women were treated with progesterone supplementation. Six women were treated with clomiphene alone, four with an increased dose, having been on clomiphene when the diagnosis was made, and two began on clomiphene because of advanced age and/or a long follicular phase. Endometrial biopsy for verification of adequate treatment was obtained in 45 of the 67 treated women, and found to be in-phase, suggesting adequate treatment in 37 (82%) (Table 12.2). One patient was sampled in the COC, but 7 of 45 (16%) biopsies clearly reflected inadequate treatment. Endometrial repair was effected by adding clomiphene in two women, increasing progesterone in three, and changing to Pergonal in one patient; one was lost to follow-up.

Table 12.2 Results of endometrial biopsy obtained during treatment

Treatment	n	Bx done	Bx on treatment			
			IP	OOP	COC	No Bx
Progesterone	54	38	32	5	1	16
Clomiphene	6	2	2	0	0	4
Both	7	5	3	2	0	2
Total	67	45	37	7	1	22

IP = in phase; OOP = out of phase; Bx = biopsy; COC = cycle of conception

In this series, 40 pregnancies were recorded, with 33 deliveries and 7 abortions, including an ectopic pregnancy (Table 12.3). Five women were biopsied in the COC, with four normal deliveries; the remaining patient aborted a fetus with trisomy 16.

Progesterone supplementation was the treatment of choice in 18 women with a history of repeated early fetal wastage diagnosed to have luteal inadequacy on at least one biopsy. Of these, 13 achieved pregnancy (Table 12.4). Eight of ten on treatment delivered, and two aborted, one with the karyotypically abnormal trisomy 16. Three became pregnant without treatment, and only one delivered, as the other two aborted.

Table 12.3 Pregnancy outcome in entire series according to choice of treatment

Treatment	n	Total pregnant	Pregnant on Rx				Pregnant after Rx discontinued			
			n	Del.	Ab.	COC	n	Del.	Ab.	COC
None	8	3	3	3	0	3	–	–	–	–
Progesterone	54	29	23	19	4	2	6	4	2	0
Clomiphene	6	2	2	2	0	0	0	0	0	0
Both	7	6	5	4	1	0	1	1*	0	0
Total	75†	40	33	28	5	5	7	5	2	0

*Treatment switched to Pergonal when endometrial defect not corrected
†Four women were lost to follow-up or received other treatment (e.g. danazol)
Del = deliveries; Ab = abortions; COC = cycle of conception; Rx = treatment

Table 12.4 Biopsy results and pregnancy outcome in women presenting with a history of early pregnancy wastage

.	Pregnant on Rx				Pregnant after Rx discontinued			
	n	Del	Ab	COC	n	Del	Ab	COC
Progesterone	17	8	1	1	3	1	2	0
Both	1		1					
Total	18	8	2	1	3	1	2	0

Del = deliveries; Ab = abortions; COC = cycle of conception; Rx = treatment

DISCUSSION

Although our results are difficult to interpret, we suggest that progesterone supplementation is an efficacious and appropriate first approach to therapy in selected patients diagnosed to have luteal inadequacy. There are few data available to verify that luteal inadequacy is an important clinical entity, or that its treatment has improved pregnancy rates. Our study, like all others in the literature, has no statistically satisfying data, contains no control groups and no randomized treatment protocol. Without a double-blind control series, unfortunately there is no substantiation of therapeutic benefit. Our study, and those mentioned earlier, are among the only ones in which progesterone supplementation has been used as the primary modality of therapy. Other authors have reported the use of bromocriptine, clomiphene, hCG stimulation, and hMG; these studies are as uncontrolled as those using progesterone alone, and also suffer from a lack of consistency in the method of diagnosis.

Several observations are important. In the first place, the biopsy obtained too early in the cycle may be misleading; eight of nine women initially found to have an in-phase biopsy were resampled in the late luteal phase revealing a clearly deranged endometrial pattern. This is not surprising as the biopsy taken later in the cycle reflects the total hormonal stimulation.

Secondly, treatment did not initially correct the endometrial pattern in 16% of patients, suggesting that follow-up biopsy during therapy is essential. Most but not all patients responded to an increased progesterone dosage. Finally, it is worthwhile to emphasize that pregnancy *rates* cannot be compared as these infertile patients had a multifactorial aetiology to explain their failure to conceive. Rather, pregnancy *outcome* has been analysed, which suggests but does not prove a benefit of progesterone supplementation.

Results of therapy may be simpler to interpret in cases of repeated early abortion, but this too is a highly controversial area. Of 120 women with repeated pregnancy wastage reported in 1951, 34 were found to have luteal phase inadequacy, and 31 delivered live babies following progesterone substitution therapy[50]. Thi Tho et al.[19] identified 23 patients with luteal phase inadequacy in a group of 100 presenting with recurrent miscarriage, and documented a 91% term-delivery rate in these patients with substitution therapy alone. Progesterone supplementation alone was used for recurrent miscarriage patients with 'double' uteri, and resulted in a 60% full-term delivery rate[35]. Finding luteal phase inadequacy associated with recurrent abortion is gratifying from the therapeutic standpoint. Yet only a randomized, double-blind, placebo-controlled treatment protocol would prove the efficacy of progesterone treatment, and there is essentially no way of performing such a study.

Even in the absence of satisfying statistical evidence, luteal phase inadequacy is being identified and treated. Every effort should be made to use consistent diagnostic criteria and a consistent approach to therapy. Collaborative studies will be required to determine the efficacy and safety of treatment with progesterone in patients with established luteal phase deficiency, because of the rarity of the defect and the necessity for randomized therapy. Patients with one or more years of infertility or a history of spontaneous early abortions should have the diagnosis established by two endometrial biopsy examinations performed premenstrually, although some exception may be made as to the need for two biopsies in certain patient categories. Treatable causes should first be sought, and only those patients treated for luteal inadequacy who fulfil established criteria. For proper statistical analysis, patients selected for therapy should be randomly assigned to either treatment or placebo groups and followed on a double-blind basis. The therapy should consist of progesterone vaginal suppositories, 25 mg twice daily, beginning 3 days after ovulation, which is assessed by means of the biphasic basal temperature chart. The progesterone suppositories should be continued until the start of menses or a positive pregnancy test is obtained. If the diagnosis, therapy and follow-up of luteal phase insufficiency could be standardized, it is expected that the safety and efficacy of this therapy might be established.

Acknowledgement

The author thanks Angela Sullivan for her secretarial expertise.

References

1. Jones, G. S. and Pourmand, K. (1962). An evaluation of etiologic factors and therapy in 555 private patients with primary infertility. *Fertil. Steril.*, **13**, 398
2. Soules, M. R., Wiebe, R. H., Aksel, S. *et al.* (1977). The diagnosis and therapy of luteal phase deficiency. *Fertil. Steril.*, **28**, 1033
3. Katayama, K. P., Ju, K-S., Manuel, M. *et al.* (1979). Computer analysis of etiology and pregnancy rate in 636 cases of primary infertility. *Am. J. Obstet. Gynecol.*, **135**, 207
4. Rosenberg, S. M., Luciano, A. A. and Riddick, D. H. (1980). The luteal phase defect: the relative frequency of, and encouraging response to, treatment with vaginal progesterone. *Fertil. Steril.*, **34**, 17
5. Balasch, J., Vanrell, J. A., Marquez, M. *et al.* (1982). Dehydrogesterone versus vaginal progesterone in the treatment of the endometrial luteal phase deficiency. *Fertil. Steril.*, **37**, 751
6. Ross, G. T. and Hillier, S. G. (1978). Luteal maturation and luteal phase defect. *Clin. Obstet. Gynecol.*, **5**, 391
7. DiZerega, G. S. and Hodgen, G. D. (1981). Luteal phase dysfunction infertility: a sequel to aberrant folliculogenesis. *Fertil. Steril.*, **35**, 489
8. DiZerega, G. S. and Hodgen, G. D. (1981). Folliculogenesis in the primate ovarian cycle. *Endocrine Rev.*, **2**, 27
9. Jones, G. E., Aksel, S. and Wentz, A. C. (1974). Serum progesterone values in the luteal phase defects: effect of chorionic gonadotropin. *Obstet. Gynecol.*, **44**, 26
10. Keller, D. W., Wiest, W. G., Askin, F. B. *et al.* (1979). Pseudocorpus luteum insufficiency: a local defect of progesterone action on endometrial stroma. *J. Clin. Endocrinol. Metab.*, **48**, 127
11. Jones, G. E. (1949). Some newer aspects of the management of infertility. *J. Am. Med. Assoc.*, **141**, 1123
12. Abraham, G. E., Maroulis, G. B. and Marshall, J. R. (1974). Evaluation of ovulation and corpus luteum function using measurements of plasma progesterone. *Obstet. Gynecol.*, **44**, 522
13. Radwanska, E., McGarrigle, H. H. G. and Swyer, G. I. M. (1976). Plasma progesterone and oestradiol estimations in the diagnosis and treatment of luteal insufficiency in menstruating infertile women. *Acta Europa, Fertil.*, **7**, 39
14. Godfrey, K. A., Aspillaga, M. O., Taylor, A. *et al.* (1981). The relation of circulating progesterone and oestradiol concentrations to the onset of menstruation. *Br. J. Obstet. Gynaecol.*, **88**, 899
15. Goldstein, D., Zuckerman, H., Harpaz, S. *et al.* (1982). Correlation between estradiol and progesterone in cycles with luteal phase deficiency. *Fertil. Steril.*, **37**, 348
16. Chatterton, R. T., Jr., Haan, J. N., Jenco, J. M. *et al.* (1982). Radioimmunoassay of pregnanediol concentrations in early morning urine specimens for assessment of luteal function in women. *Fertil. Steril.*, **37**, 361
17. Wentz, A. C. (1980). Pathophysiology of luteal phase inadequacy. In Tozzini, R. I., Reeves, G. and Pineda, R. L. (eds). *Endocrine Physiopathology of the Ovary.* pp. 257–274. (Elsevier: North-Holland Biomedical Press)
18. Wentz, A. C. (1979). Physiologic and clinical considerations in luteal phase defects. *Clin. Obstet. Gynecol.*, **22**, 169
19. Thi Tho, P. T., Byrd, J. R. and McDonough, P. G. (1979). Etiologies and subsequent reproductive performance of 100 couples with recurrent abortion. *Fertil. Steril.*, **32**, 398
20. Jones, G. S. and Delfs, E. (1951). Endocrine patterns in term pregnancies following abortions. *J. Am. Med. Assoc.*, **146**, 1212
21. Grant, A., McBride, W. G. and Moyes, J. M. (1959). Luteal phase defects in abortion. *Int. J. Fertil.*, **4**, 323
22. Garcia, J., Jones, G. S. and Wentz, A. C. (1977). The use of clomiphene citrate. *Fertil. Steril.*, **28**, 707
23. Wentz, A. C. (1980). Endometrial biopsy in the evaluation of infertility. *Fertil. Steril.*, **33**, 121
24. Del Pozo, E., Wyss, H., Tolis, G. *et al.* (1979). Prolactin and deficient luteal function. *Obstet. Gynecol.*, **53**, 282

25. Sherman, B. M., West, J. H. and Korenman, S. G. (1976). The menopausal transition: analysis of LH, FSH, estradiol, and progesterone concentrations during menstrual cycles of older women. *J. Clin. Endocrinol. Metab.*, **42**, 629
26. Driessen, F., Kremer, J., Albsbach, G. P. J. *et al.* (1980). Serum progesterone and oestradiol concentrations in women with unexplained infertility. *Br. J. Obstet. Gynaecol.*, **87**, 619
27. Shangold, M., Freeman, R., Thysen, B. *et al.* (1979). The relationship between long-distance running, plasma progesterone, and luteal phase length. *Fertil. Steril.*, **31**, 130
28. Bates, G. W., Bates, S. R. and Whitworth, N. S. (1982). Reproductive failure in women who practice weight control. *Fertil. Steril.*, **37**, 373
29. Lahteenmaki, P. and Luukkainen, T. (1978). Return of ovarian function after abortion. *Clin. Endocrinol.*, **8**, 123
30. Lahteenmaki, P., Ylostalo, P., Sipinen, S. *et al.* (1980). Return of ovulation after abortion and after discontinuation of oral contraceptives. *Fertil. Steril.*, **34**, 246
31. Brosens, I. A., Koninckx, P. R. and Corveleyn, P. A. (1976). A study of plasma progesterone, oestradiol-17β, prolactin and LH levels, and of the luteal phase appearance of the ovaries in patients with endometriosis and infertility. *Br. J. Obstet. Gynaecol.*, **85**, 246
32. Radwanska, E. and Dmowski, W. P. (1981). Luteal phase in infertile women with endometriosis. *Infertility*, **4**, 269
33. Pittaway, D. E., Maxson, W., Daniell, J. *et al.* (1983). Luteal phase defects in infertility patients with endometriosis. *Fertil. Steril.*, **39**, 712
34. Schweppe, K.-W., Dmowski, W. P. and Wynn, R. M. (1982). Ultrastructural changes in endometriotic tissue during danazol treatment. *Fertil. Steril.*, **36**, 20
35. Jones, H. W., Jr. and Wheeless, C. R. (1969). Salvage of the reproductive potential of women with anomalous development of the mullerian ducts. *Am. J. Obstet. Gynecol.*, **104**, 348
36. Wallach, E. E. (1972). The uterine factor in infertility. *Fertil. Steril.*, **23**, 138
37. Karow, W. G., Gentry, W. C., Skeels, R. F. *et al.* (1971). Endometrial biopsy in the luteal phase of the cycle of conception. *Fertil. Steril.*, **22**, 482
38. Rosenfeld, D. L. and Garcia, C.-R. (1975). Endometrial biopsy in the cycle of conception. *Fertil. Steril.*, **26**, 1088
39. Rosenberg, S. M. (1980). Inappropriateness of single midluteal progesterone for diagnosis of corpus luteum defect. *Obstet. Gynecol.*, **56**, 267
40. Rosenfeld, D. L. and Garcia, C.-R. (1976). A comparison of endometrial histology with simultaneous plasma progesterone determinations in infertile women. *Fertil. Steril.*, **27**, 1256
41. Balasch, J., Vanrell, J. A., Marquez, M. *et al.* (1982). Luteal phase in infertility: problems of evaluation. *Int. J. Fertil.*, **27**, 60
42. Abraham, G. E., Maroulis, G. B. and Marshall, J. R. (1974). Evaluation of ovulation and corpus luteum function using measurements of plasma progesterone. *Obstet. Gynecol.*, **44**, 522
43. Aksel, S. (1981). Hormonal characteristics of long cycles in fertile women. *Fertil. Steril.*, **36**, 521
44. Broom, T. J., Matthews, D. C., Cooke, I. D. *et al.* (1981). Endocrine profiles and fertility status of human menstrual cycles of varying follicular phase length. *Fertil. Steril.*, **36**, 194
45. Johansson, E. D. B. (1971). Depression of the progesterone levels in women treated with synthetic gestagens after ovulation. *Acta Endocrinol. (Kbhr.)*, **68**, 779
46. Nillius, S. J. and Johansson, E. D. B. (1971). Plasma levels of progesterone after vaginal, rectal, or intramuscular administration of progesterone. *Am. J. Obstet. Gynecol.*, **110**, 470
47. Roberts, D. K., Horbelt, D. V. and Powell, L. C., Jr. (1975). The ultrastructural response of human endometrium to medroxyprogesterone acetate. *Am. J. Obstet. Gynecol.*, **123**, 811
48. Maruffo, C. A., Casavilla, F., Van Nynatten, B. *et al.* (1974). Modifications of the human endometrial fine structure induced by low-dose progesterone therapy. *Fertil. Steril.*, **25**, 778
49. Noyes, R. W., Hertig, A. and Rock, J. (1950). Dating the endometrial biopsy. *Fertil. Steril.*, **1**, 3
50. Jones, G. S. and Delfs, E. (1951). Endocrine patterns in term pregnancies following abortions. *J. Am. Med. Assoc.*, **146**, 1212

Discussion

Koninckx	When you date the biopsy according to the onset of menstruation, how do you go about premenstrual spotting?
Wentz	I am fascinated by premenstrual spotting, which has been suggested to be a sign or symptom of luteal phase inadequacy, as I found such patients to have a 35% chance of having endometriosis as diagnosed at laparoscopy. If you ask the woman when her period began or when it is about to begin, it is surprising how accurate she can be in supplying this criterion for dating the biopsy. Also remember that the criteria of Noyes, Hertig, and Rock (*Fertil. Steril.*, **1** (1950), 3), give you much room for error in that these criteria for dating allow you a 48-hour leeway. Therefore, using this method is a very naive, simplistic approach, but it makes it unlikely to overdiagnose this entity.
L'Hermite	I have been interested in some articles which, I guess, appeared during recent years in *Fertility and Sterility*. One of them showed that there was a higher incidence of miscarriage when you performed the endometrial biopsy during the cycle of conception, but only when the endometrium was dated later than the 24th day. In consideration of this we usually tried to take a biopsy on the 24th and not the 25th day. Do you really think that taking the biopsy on the 24th instead of the 25th day could really be misleading? I would also like to comment on a question which was discussed in another paper, that there is a higher incidence of conception during cycles in which an endometrial biopsy has been performed. I am afraid that there might be a bias when the endometrial biopsy is done during the first cycle of investigation, as it may have a placebo-like effect.
	I would also like to have your opinion on whether it is possible to induce, by the mechanical stimulation of the endometrium, local changes which would make it more appropriate for nidation.
Wentz	There are perhaps four to six papers which have shown no increased incidence of miscarriage, no increased incidence of prematurity, or any untoward effect of a biopsy when it was taken in a cycle of conception. As to the second question, there are no data to suggest that the endometrial biopsy does improve the pregnancy rates, even though there are lots of individual observations.
Schneider	It is written in many textbooks that the premenstrual spotting in patients with corpus luteum insufficiency is actually a progesterone-withdrawal or progesterone-breakthrough bleeding. Do you think there is such a thing?
Wentz	I have no data on that, but premenstrual spotting was certainly not common in our series of patients with luteal phase inadequacy who were thought to have a progesterone deficiency.
Gahn	In some biopsies taken from 155 patients with infertility we found a discrepancy between the first and second one, in that the first was normal while the second was out-of-phase or vice-versa. Is this a phenomenon which can occur at some time in all women, or only in a particularly susceptible group which will also have more abortions than others?

Wentz   Obviously this question is really what we have been spending these two days talking about. I have my own bias which I shall be happy to relay. One is that luteal phase inadequacy as a cause of infertility due to recurrent miscarriage is rare; in our series about 5%. I do think that certain women under particular circumstances have repetitive cycle after cycle luteal-phase inadequacy. I also think that women, being what they are, may sporadically have an abnormal cycle for whatever aetiologic reason. The entity which we should be focusing on is the repetitive type, and not the one that occurs sporadically, perhaps for reasons such as transient hyperprolactinaemia, some form of stress, or some other aetiology.

Dallenbach   I would like to add a short remark to the question of Dr L'Hermite on the possible decidual reaction after endometrial biopsy. We have performed a study precisely on that subject. Our observation was that mechanical stimulation of the endometrium does induce a decidual reaction which can occur as early as the second or third day after ovulation, whereas under normal conditions you do not expect it before the last week of the cycle. This reaction, however, does not enhance, but rather prevents, the implantation of the blastocyst, because once the decidua has been formed, the blastocyst cannot implant any more. This is, incidentally, one of the effects of intrauterine devices.

Keller   Dr Wentz, do you have any experience with hCG-stimulation of the corpus luteum?

Wentz   Yes and no, but I do not have any data to present. It is unusual that we use hCG as a primary treatment for an inadequate luteal phase. We use hCG in conjunction with clomiphene under certain circumstances. Occasionally I use hCG when the patient might have a luteinized, unruptured follicle in order to produce another LH-surge to promote prostaglandin synthesis and the formation of a stigma. I will, however, take you back to the patient described by Dr Georgeanna Jones many years ago in an early publication, who had had a history of nine early miscarriages. She was diagnosed as having luteal phase inadequacy by biopsy criteria. Dr Jones treated her with hCG supplementation in relatively high doses to see if the corpus luteum could indeed be rescued. The patient became pregnant and again miscarried. Only when the patient was given progesterone supplementation was she able to carry the pregnancy. This is perhaps the only documented case of a resistant corpus luteum that is in the literature, probably resistant because of a receptor or enzyme defect, but nevertheless inappropriate to respond to relatively high doses of hCG, exogenous or endogenous. It needs to be re-emphasized because of my bias that the implantation site is important. Though progesterone may have many effects in the luteal phase, its primary target organ is the endometrium. We felt, therefore, that we can bypass much of the corpus luteum inadequacy by going directly to the target organ inadequacy.

Taubert   We have treated a good number of patients with hCG and were careful to give the first injection after the rise of the basal temperature curve. We are all aware that one can raise serum progesterone levels quite nicely by doing this, but our results were disappointing. When we used dydrogesterone, 37.5% of the patients with luteal phase inadequacy became pregnant as compared to 18.9% who received hCG.

Wentz   I think one of the major problems we have in talking is that we all want to look at pregnancy rates. We cannot discuss that now, so I want to ask you, was the endometrium repaired?

Taubert   We have not followed this in all of our patients who did not conceive, but we can confirm your data in that the endometrium of most of the patients who did not conceive and underwent a repeat biopsy remained out-of-phase irrespective of the type of therapy we used.

Breckwoldt   Do you think recurrent abortion is primarily a genetic problem?

Wentz	Obviously, 50–60% of miscarriages are indeed due to random rearrangement of the chromosomes. There is perhaps also a situation in which there could be corpus luteum inadequacy on the basis of some form of genetic problem. That is a little bit hard to recombine, but we have to remember that there is a cross-talk between the implantation site and the corpus luteum.
Breckwoldt	I am not quite convinced because treatment ought to be much more efficient if your idea were correct. My feeling is that the fate of a pregnancy is determined at the moment of conception. If the chromosomes are properly arranged there will be a healthy pregnancy which will regulate its own requirements. When, however, the development of the oocyte is disturbed, spontaneous abortion will ensue.
Schweppe	We can confirm your finding of a remarkable percentage of out-of-phase endometria even if the plasma levels of estradiol and progesterone are in the normal range. This is our reason to stress the importance of a follow-up biopsy. But what are the consequences for therapy? Do you recommend increasing the dosage or the duration of progesterone treatment, or do you think that the consequence should be to change the therapeutic regimen?
Wentz	If the patient has been on progesterone supplementation alone, we have increased the dose of progesterone. If she has been on clomiphene alone, we have ordinarily added progesterone supplementation. If the patient has been on clomiphene plus progesterone, and still has an out-of-phase biopsy, we have a problem.
Musil	Progesterone was your first compound of choice, but you also showed on your illustration that it has very unfavourable kinetics. Do you think that you would have better, or at least equally good, results with Depo-Provera?
Wentz	Here we have a dilemma that is perhaps medico-legally dictated. Some progestational agents are certainly teratogenic. The only teratogenic effect of progesterone is to cause an increased incidence of hypospadias if given somewhat later in pregnancy and in higher doses. Although Provera has a relatively benign history, it is very much on the list of drugs that are opposed by the FDA. If, however, you studied the endometrium of Provera-treated patients, you would find an increased chance of glandular–stromal disparity, i.e. an increased stromal response over that of the glands. The inappropriate endometrial pattern, and the fact that Provera is very much opposed by the FDA, has led us away from using Provera as a progestational supplement. The kinetics of progesterone are indeed such that it does disappear from the circulation very rapidly. But most patients do well with b.i.d. progesterone suppositories, and get a relatively good level over the 24 hours of the day.
Dallenbach	I have to support what Dr Wentz said. The progestational agents, particularly of the nortestosterone group, but also the 17α-hydroxyprogesterone derivatives, affect the endometrium in a very different way from the natural progesterone. As a consequence, they should not be used for this type of therapy.
Keller	It has become quite common to administer steroid hormones vaginally. Could you say something about acceptability, and do the patients not complain about vaginal discharge?
Wentz	Vaginal discharge is not a common complaint. The major side-effect of progesterone supplementation is the problem of poverty. This medication is in the hands of a pharmacist, who makes it so expensive that most patients stop it after 2–3 months of use, simply on the basis of expense. For that reason we have that albeit small group of patients who conceived after they stopped medication for some reason.
Taubert	Did you follow these patients with PAP smears, to discover whether the high concentration of progesterone does anything to the cervical epithelium?

DISCUSSION

Wentz

We have not followed up with PAP smears, but over the many years of experience with progesterone in several institutions I have not found that there has been any suggestion of an abnormality. That is a very weak kind of statement, but having been at Johns Hopkins I suspect something would have been detected because of the epidemiological projects which had been done there. The therapy is begun when one is assured that the temperature has risen, and I stay away from the term 'ovulation', because I do not know when ovulation occurred. We feel that for every patient the temperature chart is necessary, and for every patient there is a temperature above which one can be relatively assured that full ovulation has occurred. For most women this is 97.8 °F (36.5 °C) for at least three consecutive days, then the patients begin the therapy, and it is continued until menses begins. If menses does not occur, pregnancy is very likely. We have not seen a continuation of the luteal phase under progesterone treatment alone. What we wish to avoid is the following: if a patient begins the progesterone supplementation too early before full ovulation has occurred, then, because of an increase in progesterone, she will inhibit ovulation.

L'Hermite

There is active, micronized progesterone available in some European countries, and in Germany also percutaneous progesterone gel. This might be more agreeable to use than vaginal suppositories.

13
Treatment of luteal insufficiency by induction of ovulation

V. INSLER, G. HOLCBERG, D. GOLDSTEIN,
J. LEVY AND G. POTASHNIK

INTRODUCTION

Corpus luteum insufficiency (CLI) (synonyms: luteal phase defect, inadequate luteal phase, short luteal phase, luteal insufficiency) is a rather rare finding. Israel[1] reported that 3.5% of 904 infertile women showed this pathology. Jones and Pourmand[2] estimated the frequency of CLI to be 3.7%. Gillam[3] found that 10.7% of infertile patients had endometrial inadequacy. In women with repeated abortions Jones and Delfs[4] found a much higher incidence of luteal insufficiency (35%). According to Taubert[5] this pathology occurs in 3–10% of infertile patients. Perusal of 600 files from our Infertility Clinic revealed the diagnosis of corpus luteum insufficiency in 30 cases (4.3%).

Inadequate luteal phase may also be iatrogenic, complicating induction of ovulation[6-8]. Recently, hyperprolactinaemia has also been indicated as a possible cause of CLI[9-11].

The diagnosis of CLI is a somewhat controversial issue. Georgeanna Jones[12] suggested endometrial biopsy (EB) as an adequate diagnostic tool. Indeed, endometrial specimens can be dated very accurately, enabling their placement within a normal 28 days' cycle scale with an error not exceeding 2 days[13]. Abraham et al.[14] and Lehmann and Bettendorf[15] advocated plasma progesterone assays (three estimations during the luteal phase) as a convenient and accurate diagnostic method for assessment of corpus luteum function. Cooke and Lambadarios[16] suggested a combination of basal body temperature records (BBT), well-timed endometrial biopsy and hormonal assays as the most feasible and reliable diagnostic means. Indeed, such a combination might overcome the inaccuracy of BBT, the inconvenience of repeated endometrial biopsies and the cost of daily steroid assays.

The aim of the present study was to assess the luteal function in 12 infertile women with previous clinical diagnosis of CLI, and to try to improve this function by induction of ovulation using gonadotropin-releasing hormone (GnRH), clomiphene citrate or human menopausal gonadotropin (hMG).

MATERIAL AND METHODS

Twelve women were elected for this study. All were infertile for at least 2 years and none received fertility-promoting treatment within 3 months preceding the study. All were previously diagnosed as having corpus luteum insufficiency according to the following criteria:

(a) sustained high phase of basal temperature not exceeding 10 days;
(b) plasma progesterone between 3.0 and 9.0 ng/ml on two examinations performed at least 2 days apart between the 5th and 10th day following the BBT nadir.

The diagnosis of CLI was established when the above findings were present either in two consecutive cycles or in the majority of cycles.

Other pertinent clinical data are listed below:

The mean age of the women was 31.2 years (median 31½, range 27–38). Seven patients had primary and five secondary infertility, none had had repeated abortions.

The duration of infertility was: 2 years in two women; 3 years in four patients; 4 years in two couples and 5, 7, 9 and 10 years each in one patient.

In three couples the male partners had mild oligo-terato-astheno-spermia (OTA) and in three others severe OTA or azoospermia. In the latter couples induction of ovulation was accompanied by *AID*. None of the females has had tubal occlusion or other severe mechanical disturbance of fertility.

All women participating in this study had an evaluation cycle followed by one or two treatment cycles. The evaluation cycle consisted of daily basal temperature record, late luteal phase or premenstrual endometrial biopsy, repeated examinations of the uterine cervix and its mucus (expressed as the cervical score according to Insler *et al.*[17]) as well as six estimations of FSH, LH, 17β-estradiol, prolactin and progesterone. Plasma prolactin, LH and FSH concentrations were determined using commercial radioimmunoassay kits supplied by Diagnostic Product Corporation (DPC) of California, USA. For radioimmunoassay of progesterone and 17β-estradiol antibodies from Radioassay Systems Laboratory (California, USA) and radioactive steroids from Amersham (England) were employed. Plasma was extracted prior to the steroid assays.

In all hormone measurements the intra-assay and inter-assay coefficient of variation did not exceed 4.1% and 9.2% respectively.

Blood for hormonal assays was drawn every 2–4 days starting between the 8th and 12th cycle day. It was hoped that this regime, simple enough to be applicable in clinical practice, will nevertheless cover fairly well the periovulatory and luteal phases of the cycle.

The treatments applied were: clomiphene citrate, GnRH and hMG. Clomiphene was used in a standard dose of 100 mg per day for 5 days starting on the 5th cycle day.

GnRH was applied in a pulsatile manner using an indwelling intravenous catheter and a computerized pump (generously supplied by Ferring, West Germany) that delivered 20 μg of native hormone every 90 min. The treatment was started on the 5th cycle day and continued until 2 or 3 days following presumed ovulation and was then supplemented with three injections of 10 000 units of human chorionic gonadotropin (hCG) on consecutive days, starting on the 3rd–6th luteal day. The GnRH treatment was discontinued if ovulation failed to occur within 21 days of therapy.

Human menopausal gonadotropin was given in combination with hCG using the individually adjusted treatment scheme (Insler and Lunenfeld[18]).

The above-mentioned treatments were each given to five patients. Three women received both clomiphene and hMG therapy. The examination regime during the treatment cycles was similar to that of the control cycles with two minor deviations: the frequency of mucus and estrogen examinations was higher in treatment cycles (particularly during hMG therapy); endometrial biopsy was performed during the first hours of menstruation in order to minimize the psychological impact of an intrauterine procedure in women trying to conceive. For this reason EB was carried out only in eight of the 15 treatment cycles.

RESULTS AND DISCUSSION

Cycle evaluation

The mean overall cycle length was 28 days. Two patients had a short cycle of 25 days and 10 women exhibited a cycle of normal duration (25–35 days). Although all the 12 patients were previously diagnosed as luteal insufficiency, not all exhibited on cycle evaluation a significantly shortened high-temperature phase (Table 13.1). In fact, seven women had a luteal phase of 13 ± 2 days, one patient had a monophasic cycle and only four women showed a typical short luteal phase of 10 days or less. In eight patients the presence of LH peak could be assumed since one of the six assays produced a result at least twice as high as the mean value of all assays. In four other women the LH peak was either absent or not detected because of the timing of examinations.

In five women a preovulatory E_2 peak could be presumed to exist (one value exceeded by 100% the mean of all assays) and in seven patients it was either missed or lacking.

Both LH and E_2 peak were present in four women and absent in three others. In five instances one assay (LH or E_2) showed a possible peak value while the other failed to do so.

In nine women progesterone assays during the luteal phase were low (3–9 ng/ml) and in three patients at least two out of six progesterone assays showed values equal to or exceeding 10 ng/ml (Table 13.1).

In five women transient (spiking) hyperprolactinaemia was evident (two or more of the six assays exceeding 20 ng/ml).

Table 13.1 Length of sustained high-temperature phase and hormonal assays in patients previously diagnosed as CLI

Case No.	Length of luteal phase (days)	LH Peak*	E₂ Peak*	Progesterone
1	11	no	no	low
2	12	yes	yes	low
3	14	no	yes	low
4	10	yes	no	low
5	monophasic	yes	no	high†
6	14	no	no	low
7	12	yes	no	low
8	10	yes	yes	low
9	15	yes	yes	high†
10	11	yes	no	low
11	9	yes	yes	low
12	9	no	no	high†

*At least one assay exceeding by 100% the mean value of all examinations
†At least 2 values equal to or exceeding 10 ng/ml

All patients, except for two, showed a rise and a subsequent decrease of the cervical score, as expected in ovulatory cycles. The endometrial dating corresponded to the day of the cycle in one woman only (Table 13.2). This patient had a luteal phase of 15 days, evidence of both LH and E₂ peaks and progesterone levels compatible with ovulation. In five patients the EB was out of phase by 2–4 days, in three cases by 4–6 days and in three women the discrepancy between the endometrial dating and menstrual cycle day exceeded 6 days. None of the biopsies showed proliferative endometrium.

The above data enabled us to form the following conclusions: luteal insufficiency is not necessarily a persistent feature appearing in all cycles of the same patient. It may be interspersed between apparently ovulatory and

Table 13.2 Comparison of endometrial dating and timing of biopsy

Case No.	Endometrial dating	Biopsy on cycle day	Difference
1	18–19	24	−5
2	18–19	25	−6
3	19–20	27	−7
4	18–19	23	−4
5	17–18	25	−7
6	25–26	23	+2
7	18–19	23	−4
8	24–25	27	−2
9	24–25	24	0
10	19–20	24	−4
11	18–19	27	−8
12	19–20	26	−6

completely anovulatory cycles. In this small selected group of patients previously diagnosed as CLI at least one cycle was probably ovulatory and one other anovulatory.

The diagnosis of luteal insufficiency may be difficult. Daily assays of gonadotropins and steroids would undoubtedly be sufficient for an accurate diagnosis, but are costly and inconvenient to the patient. Moreover, even a highly accurate diagnosis established in one cycle may not necessarily be representative of other cycles in the same patient.

We attempted to overcome some of these difficulties by using a standard array of examinations consisting of BBT record, cervical score estimations, endometrial biopsy and six hormonal assays so timed that three would be taken around the time of presumed ovulation and three during the luteal phase. The examinations during the evaluation cycle were scheduled on the basis of previous BBT records.

As expected, LH and E_2 assays, within the regime employed, were of little value in confirming or disproving the diagnosis of luteal insufficiency. In 10 out of 12 cases these assays were either contradictory one to the other or in disagreement with other parameters such as the duration of thermal shift or progesterone levels (Table 13.1).

The BBT records seemed to be a rather unreliable tool in indicating luteal insufficiency (Table 13.3). Among the 12 patients examined, only four exhibited a clear-cut short luteal phase. Both progesterone assays and endometrial biopsy seemed to be much better indicators of luteal insufficiency. According to the former 11 out of 12 cycles examined, and according to the latter nine of the cycles, would be diagnosed as CLI.

According to our data a combination of BBT, endometrial biopsy and progesterone assays (two or three during the luteal phase) would be both

Table 13.3 Length of sustained high-temperature phase, endometrial dating and progesterone levels in women previously diagnosed as CLI

Case No.	Length of luteal phase (days)	Endometrial biopsy	Progesterone
5	monophasic	OOP	high*
11	9	OOP	low
12	9	OOP	high*
4	10	OOP	low
8	10	OOP	low
1	11	OOP	low
10	11	OOP	low
2	12	OOP	low
7	12	OOP	low
3	14	OOP	low
6	14	OOP	low
9	15	corr.	high*

OOP = endometrium out of phase by at least 2 days; corr. = endometrium dating corresponding to cycle day
*At least two values equal to or exceeding 10 ng/ml

reliable and convenient for diagnosis of luteal insufficiency. The diagnosis is established when two of the above three indicators are abnormal. Using these criteria 10 cycles would be diagnosed as luteal insufficiency, one cycle (Case No. 9) would be considered as normal ovulatory and one (Case No. 5) would be regarded as anovulatory (Table 13.3).

Results of treatment

Of the 15 treatment cycles only 12 were analysed. In three others either EB or progesterone assays were unavailable. The treatment employed was induction of ovulation using GnRH, clomiphene or hMG/hCG. The rationale was 2-fold: to induce a well-timed ovulation by either of the three agents and, by using the last two, to produce multiple ovulations in the hope that at least one of the corpora lutea will function properly.

DiZerega and Hodgen[19, 20] reported that inadequate follicular maturation due to a relative FSH deficit may be the cause of CLI. Thus, induction of ovulation providing an appropriate FSH and LH stimulation throughout the cycle should produce both a normal ovulation and an adequate corpus luteum.

As judged by the above criteria (two out of three parameters normal). GnRH therapy resulted in normalization of the cycle in three of the four trials. One woman conceived (Table 13.4). Clomiphene therapy produced a

Table 13.4 Comparison of luteal function parameters in control and treatment cycles

	Control cycle			Treatment cycle		
Case No.	Length of luteal phase (days)	Endometrial biopsy dating	Progesterone	Length of luteal phase (days)	Endometrial biopsy dating	Progesterone
			GnRH			
1	11	OOP	low	20	—	low†
6	14	OOP	low	13	corr.	high*
7	12	OOP	low	10	OOP	high*
8	10	OOP	low	14	corr.	high*
10	11	OOP	low	Pregnancy		
			Clomiphene			
2	12	OOP	low	15	corr.	high*
3	14	OOP	low	10	corr.	low
5	monoph.	OOP	high*	Pregnancy		
11	9	OOP	low	12	—	low†
12	9	OOP	high*	17	—	high*
			hMG/hCG			
2	12	OOP	low	14	—	low†
3	14	OOP	low	10	corr.	low
4	10	OOP	low	18	corr.	low
9	15	corr.	high*	14	corr.	high*
11	9	OOP	low	Pregnancy		

†Cycle deleted in final analysis. Other abbreviations and symbols as in Table 13.3

normal cycle in three out of four cases and one of the patients conceived (Table 13.4). Induction of ovulation with hMG/hCG produced an apparently normal cycle in three instances (including one pregnancy). One cycle showed a corpus luteum insufficiency (Table 13.4).

It seems, therefore, that induction of ovulation is a fairly efficient tool for improving inadequate luteal function. Nine of the 12 treatment cycles (75%) showed a presumably normal luteal phase. Since in these women the majority of previously evaluated cycles and 10 of the 12 cycles analysed in detail were considered as insufficient with regard to the corpus luteum function, this improvement seems to be of clinical significance. The three conceptions occurred in women with primary infertility of 3, 4 and 9 years' duration. One additional finding should be mentioned here. Transient (spiking) hyperprolactinaemia was found in control cycles of five women. In four of them ovulation-inducing treatment corrected the CLI, and in one the therapy resulted in a sustained high-temperature phase of 17 days but this cycle was not included in final analysis because hormonal assays and/or EB were not available. Two of these patients conceived under treatment. Application of GnRH resulted in a significant increase of prolactin levels ($p < 0.05$). The mean prolactin level in control cycles was 15.42 ± 0.19 ng/ml (SEM). In the same women GnRH therapy produced a mean prolactin level of 23.03 ± 1.91 ng/ml (SEM). However, despite the elevated prolactin, in three out of four GnRH treatment cycles the corpus luteum function was considered to be adequate and one resulted in pregnancy.

These findings indicate that mild transient hyperprolactinaemia (sporadic spikes of 25–50 ng/ml) is not incompatible with normal corpus luteum function.

This study enabled us to form the following conclusions:

(1) CLI may not necessarily be a permanent phenomenon occurring in all cycles of a particular woman.
(2) Diagnosis of CLI may be difficult. Fully accurate and reliable diagnostic methods are too complicated and/or expensive to be applied in a large number of patients or in several consecutive cycles in the same woman. Simple measures, such as BBT, cervical score and single progesterone assays, are not reliable enough for diagnosis. It seems that a combination of BBT, endometrial biopsy and two well-timed progesterone assays may serve as a convenient and reasonably reliable diagnostic tool. The diagnosis of CLI is made when two of the above three parameters are abnormal.
(3) Induction of ovulation using clomiphene citrate, GnRH or hMG/hCG is efficient in improving inadequate luteal function.

References

1. Israel, S. L. (1967). *Diagnosis and Treatment of Menstrual Disorders and Sterility* (5th edn). (New York: Harper and Row)
2. Jones, G. E. S. and Pourmand, K. (1962). An evaluation of etiologic factors and therapy in 555 private patients with primary infertility. *Fertil. Steril.*, **13**, 398

3. Gillam, J. S. (1955). Study of inadequate secretion phase endometrium. *Fertil. Steril.*, **6**, 18
4. Jones, G. E. S. and Delfs, E. (1951). Endometrium patterns in term pregnancies following abortions. *J. Am. Med. Assoc.*, **146**, 1212
5. Taubert, H. D. (1978). Luteal phase insufficiency. In Keller, P. J. (ed.). *Contributions to Gynecology and Obstetrics.* p. 108. (Basel: Karger)
6. Murray, M. and Osmond-Clarke, F. (1971). Pregnancy results following treatment with clomiphene citrate. *J. Obstet. Gynaecol. Br. Commonw.*, **78**, 1108
7. Insler, V. and Lunenfeld, B. (1983). *Diagnose und Therapie endokriner Fertilitätsstörungen der Frau.* p. 103. (Berlin: Grosse Verlag)
8. Jones, H. W. (1983). Factors influencing implantation and maintenance of pregnancy following embryo transfer. In Beier, H. M. and Lindner, H. R. (eds). *Fertilization of the Human Egg in vitro.* pp. 294–306. (Berlin: Springer)
9. Del Pozo, E., Wyss, H., Alcaniz, J., Camapana, A. and Naftolin, F. (1979): Prolactin and deficient luteal function. *Obstet. Gynecol.*, **54**, 282
10. Seppälä, M., Hirvonen, E. and Ranta, T. (1976). Hyperprolactinemia and luteal insufficiency. *Lancet*, **1**, 229
11. Mühlenstedt, D., Bohnet, H. G., Hanker, J. P. and Schneider, H. P. G. (1978). Short luteal phase and prolactin. *Int. J. Fertil.*, **23**, 213
12. Jones, G. (1968). Luteal phase defects. In Behrman, S. J. and Kistner, R. W. (eds). *Progress in Infertility.* p. 299. (Boston: Little, Brown)
13. Noyes, R. W., Hertig, A. and Rock, J. (1950). Dating the endometrial biopsy. *Fertil. Steril.*, **1**, 3
14. Abraham, G. E., Maroulis, G. B. and Marshall, J. R. (1974). Evaluation of ovulation and corpus luteum function using measurements of plasma progesterone. *Obstet. Gynecol.*, **44**, 552
15. Lehmann, F. and Bettendorf, G. (1981). The endocrine shift from a normal cycle to anovulation. In Insler, V. and Bettendorf, G. (eds). *Advances in Diagnosis and Treatment of Infertility.* p. 105. (New York: Elsevier/North Holland)
16. Cooke, I. D. and Lambadarios, C. (1974). The endometrium. In Cooke, J. D. (ed.): *Clinics in Obstetrics and Gynaecology.* Vol. 1, p. 369. (London: Saunders)
17. Insler, V., Melmed, H., Eichenrenner, I., Serr, D. M. and Lunenfeld, B. (1972). The cervical score – a simple semi-quantitative method for monitoring of the menstrual cycle. *Int. J. Gynecol. Obstet.*, **10**, 223
18. Insler, V. and Lunenfeld, B. (1974). Application of human gonadotropins for induction of ovulation. In Campos Da Paz, A., Hasegawa, T., Notake, Y. and Hayashi, M. (eds). *Human Reproduction.* p. 25. (Tokyo: Igaku Shoin)
19. DiZerega, G. S. and Hodgen, G. (1981). Follicular phase treatment of luteal phase dysfunction. *Fertil. Steril.*, **35**, 428
20. DiZerega, G. S. and Hodgen, G. (1981). Luteal phase dysfunction: a sequel to aberrant folliculogenesis. *Fertil. Steril.*, **35**, 489

Discussion

Keller	Before I open the paper of Dr Insler for discussion I would like to state that it is of utmost importance to end these discussions with some recommendation on how we are going to treat luteal phase inadequacy. You made it quite clear that you would prefer ovulation-inducing agents to all others. Did I understand that right?
Insler	No, I did not say that. We used ovulation-induction because we thought it was a logical approach. I did not imply that any other kind of treatment has to be less efficient, although in clinical practice we use ovulation-induction and not supplementation with hCG or progesterone.
Breckwoldt	I think the remarks of Dr Insler fit very well into our concept, that follicular development should be stimulated in order to normalize luteal function. I must admit, however, that we are not as satisfied with the pregnancy rate as we would have wished. As there are very interesting animal experiments which point out the essential rôle of FSH for the early follicular phase, we will adhere to the therapeutic approach of stimulating follicular development until somebody has a better idea.
Rothchild	Hodgen and DiZerega could show that inhibiting FSH caused luteal insufficiency, but treating the animals with FSH did not restore luteal function.
Bettendorf	I think we should remember that we have had the means to stimulate ovarian function for nearly 25 years. Before that there was only the possibility of supplementing progesterone. It has at least been my experience that supplementation with progestational agents is not effective. When we calculated the pregnancy rate for the last 10 years obtained by treating women with luteal phase inadequacy both with hMG/hCG and clomiphene, we found the number of pregnancies to be much lower as compared to the treatment of amenorrhoeic women. Even though we certainly can improve the condition, we still have not found the proper way of treating luteal phase inadequacy.
Lehmann	I wonder why nobody has yet asked the question as to how sure one can be that ovulation actually takes place in a particular cycle. If it should fail to do so, any type of supplementary treatment would be doomed to failure. On the other hand, if one is reasonably sure that the egg has been released, e.g. by means of sonographic examination, the administration of progesterone would be logical. Moreover, I would like to emphasize that there are patients who continue having insufficient cycles even though they have received ovulation-inducers. How are you going to approach this problem?
Insler	You have to realize that we are dealing with a 'big bag' containing a lot of quite different things. When we disregard women with the LUF syndrome and the PCO syndrome, we are faced with a group of patients who presumably ovulate but do not conceive. It should not come as a surprise that the results of ovulation-induction in this group of patients are much worse than in amenorrhoeic women. In the latter we are conducting a type of replacement therapy which is almost completely under our control. In women with luteal phase inadequacy we interfere with the cycle.

On the other hand, there is an advantage to ovulation-induction therapy, as it has been shown by Hodgen that added FSH brings about the development of more follicles which are late, ready for selection of the dominant one. That means you can raise more than one generation of follicles in one cycle, one of which eventually will ovulate. If more than one ovulates, there is a chance that only one of them will result in an inadequate corpus luteum. I am still not convinced that the treatment with progesterone is more logical or better, except in the case of patients who have been known to abort habitually.

Rothchild Regardless of what the causes might be, the crucial question is if treatment is changing the endometrium in a way which would make a pregnancy possible. Only the progesterone treatment is attacking this problem directly, and it does not make any difference whether it is doing that because of an ovulation defect or a follicular phase defect. That is all the patient wants, and that is all the doctor wants. There is as yet no comparison between the effects of clomiphene, GnRH treatment, and hMG treatment on the one hand, and the progesterone treatment on the other. They are two entirely different ball parks. And that is why I cannot argue with you as to why and how something works, as long as you get good results. Stick to it, even though you do not know how it works.

Dallenbach-Hellweg I quite agree with what Dr Rothchild just said. It is possible to recognize the progesterone deficiency in the endometrium by means of the disparity between glandular and stromal differentiation. This explains, I believe, that we obtain better results with replacement therapy as compared to clomiphene treatment. In addition, if we follow the tenet of *nil nocere*, we should at first try to substitute what is missing in the luteal phase, and if that fails, there is time to resort to more drastic types of treatment. If there is, however, a co-ordinated form of delayed endometrial development, the approach described by Dr Insler appears preferable.

Insler The induction of ovulation appears to be much more efficient in rendering the endometrium in-phase than in causing pregnancy.

Breckwoldt Is the proper secretory transformation of the endometrium so critical? How do we explain the extrauterine pregnancy? The blastocyst seems to be capable of implanting in areas devoid of secretory endometrium!

Dallenbach-Hellweg I wish I had an answer for that. But we do know that the blastocyst will not implant in an endometrium which has not been properly prepared to receive the fertilized ovum.

Geisthövel Is it right that you used 20 μg GnRH per pulse? This would be less than Leyendecker used in amenorrhoeic patients.

Insler It is actually very high, because we used 20 μg GnRH per pulse. We tried the dose of 5 μg per pulse and found that it did not work.

Runnebaum It has become clear to me during these two days of discussion that the type of corpus luteum insufficiency we have been talking about does not exist. There are no clinical data to differentiate between a normal corpus luteum and an abnormal one. How can we find the right way of treating this entity, if we basically do not know what we are talking about, and do not have any biochemical parameters which would help us to differentiate? Moreover, any type of treatment which has as yet been discussed has been applied in every possible order for the past 15–20 years, and all these resulted in a pregnancy rate between 20% and 30%. Finally, if Dr Wentz states that pregnancy rate is no criterion either, I have to conclude that we have to meet again for a continuation of this discussion.

Section 4
General Discussion

General Discussion

Schneider

In order to give the general discussion some sort of structure, we should try at first to re-evaluate what has been said about pathogenesis. Thereafter, we should attempt to define as closely as possible what we consider corpus luteum insufficiency to be. The next part of the discussion should be devoted to diagnostic aspects, and this should lead to a discussion of the problems of therapy. As Prof. Rothchild has been covering the topic of pathogenesis in depth, I would like to ask him for a comment on what he considers as new aspects and insights.

Rothchild

I shall try to be very brief. What we have seen in these papers has not changed my mind on how little we know about what causes a corpus luteum to be inadequate. There is without doubt something like an insufficient corpus luteum, and it is reflected in the duration and the total amount of progesterone secreted. Again, probably the most important causes for this lie in the development of a follicle to the point of maturation, and its ability to induce an adequate LH-surge, and to respond to it. I have to emphasize again the experiments of Terranova *et al.* (*Biol. Reprod.*, **26**, 721; 1982), and point out that what we sometimes call an inadequate corpus luteum is probably not an ovulated follicle but a follicle that has gone in atresia, and is secreting progesterone from a luteinized theca. I do not know how to differentiate between these.

Unless one knows the cause of the inadequate corpus luteum specifically, the only way we can treat the problem is empirically, and this is what we are doing now. Finding the cause of each instance of disturbed corpus luteum function is extremely important, and there are many causes. I have left out in my presentation some of the things which may be involved, such as the fact that LH might be luteolytic just as luteotrophic, the observation that an inadequate corpus luteum might lead to another inadequate one, that the relationship of prostaglandins to progesterone in the corpus luteum may be disturbed for some reason or another, and the role of intra-follicular factors or factors in the follicular fluid which Dr Daume spoke about. But really the most difficult question of all nobody, including myself, has an answer to: how to go about identifying any one of these or other factors that may be involved, and there might be an enormous number in addition to the ones I have mentioned.

We know, for instance, that the main source of cholesterol for steroidogenesis in the corpus luteum is not the cholesterol it makes itself but the cholesterol it receives from the general circulation in the form of lipoproteins. These have to bind to the corpus luteum, have to be internalized, to be used and metabolized. Any one of the processes, if it went wrong, could lead to an inadequate secretion of progesterone. I come back to that again, if you get 50% of your patients pregnant by treating them with progesterone, what difference does it make?

187

Schneider   You mentioned in your paper that corpus luteum insufficiency could also be some sort of transitional stage between normal ovulation and full-blown anovulation. As the final pathway for inducing follicular maturation is LH-RH, it could just be nothing but a relative or gradual insufficiency of LH-RH secretion which, in some cases, renders a woman's corpus luteum insufficient, and in other circumstances makes her anovulatory or amenorrhoeic. We are possibly dealing with the reverse of the ontogeny of the menstrual cycle in adolescence.

Rothchild   But it is not the only answer. You can treat all patients with presumed corpus luteum insufficiency with LH-RH, and you should get a certain incidence of cures. That does not, however, mean that the patient at the particular moment is having an insufficient corpus luteum or is just about to have one.

Even progesterone treatment is probably not the whole answer because Cooke or someone else has pointed out that it is not just an insufficiency of progesterone, but that estrogen may also be involved in the transformation of the endometrium in a proper way. That is well known, and just correcting it with progesterone may give some results, but they could possibly even be better if progesterone is combined with estrogen at the proper dose.

I cannot say much more about pathogenesis except to state that the corpus luteum is probably the most complicated organ in the whole body, and there are a million things which can go wrong with it.

Koninckx   It is one of the difficulties in defining corpus luteum insufficiency that normally we do not see 'pure' cases, as they are rare. The second point is, I do not think it is absolutely necessary for every woman with corpus luteum insufficiency to have this condition in every cycle. The situation may be compared to immunological infertility: the higher the anti-sperm titre is, the less likely is the woman to conceive. As the titre may change, it is not impossible that she eventually will become pregnant.

Schneider   What is the proof for ovulation really having taken place in a case of corpus luteum inadequacy?

Insler   In one word: none, unless the patient conceives or it is possible to demonstrate the stigma at laparoscopy. That means that we usually have to depend on circumstantial evidence, and should really not speak of ovulatory but presumably ovulatory cycles.

Schneider   It was Lehmann's argument that we are dealing mainly with the anovulation syndrome rather than corpus luteum inadequacy.

Insler   This is certainly the worst group for ovulation induction as far as the pregnancy rate is concerned. If the infertility were really due to anovulation we could expect better results with ovulation induction.

Dallenbach-Hellweg   I think we can exclude anovulation from what we are talking about by the endometrial biopsy. In the presence of an unruptured, luteinized follicle the endometrium would appear normal. In a real case of anovulation we would find a proliferative endometrium, and not a deficient secretory one.

Schneider   I wonder if there is somebody in the audience who would uphold the idea that you can diagnose ovulation by means of an endometrial biopsy?

Dallenbach-Hellweg   You can distinguish between an endometrium which is under the influence of a persistent follicle with sporadic luteinization, and a deficient secretory phase following ovulation.

Rothchild   But you cannot differentiate between a luteinized, unruptured follicle and a corpus luteum with rupture by endometrial biopsy.

Dallenbach-Hellweg   Well, I can.

Taubert   Have you studied endometria obtained by biopsy a few days after a laparoscopy, when a stigma could be identified, and a high level of progesterone was demonstrated in the peritoneal fluid? If you have such data, I would accept your claim.

Dallenbach-Hellweg	I do not have that kind of material, but we do have such correlations for anovulatory cycles, and also for endometria which show only abortive secretion due to sporadic luteinization within a persistent follicle.
Taubert	I would like to advise caution with respect to the interpretation of the basal body temperature, as I just had the experience of finding at laparoscopy a fresh corpus luteum with a rupture in a patient with a persistently monophasic basal body temperature even though there was a progesterone level of 14 ng/ml in the peripheral blood.
Rothchild	There is at least one report in the literature claiming that there is a higher association between the luteinized, unruptured follicle and the inadequate luteal phase than one would expect ordinarily. Though the LUF syndrome can result in a corpus luteum which is undifferentiable from a normal one, it can be associated with an inadequate one as well, and there is no reason why it should not be.
Wentz	All we heard at this stage of the general discussion was again a problem with diagnosis. If one bases the diagnosis on the endometrial target organ the pathogenesis could be sought in two areas. On one hand, there may be a decrease in progesterone output or an abnormal estradiol/progesterone ratio, and this would cover a multitude of pre-ovulatory determinants. Similarly, if one defines a luteal phase inadequacy on the basis of endometrial target organ problems, there is also a whole multitude of entities. Moreover, there may also be factors which could cause problems with implantation, and these are not necessarily associated with a progesterone defect.

In order to benefit the patients in terms of implantation we have preferred to go to the target organ and not to spend as much time massaging, if you will, the corpus luteum. What we have not heard is if there is any true necessity for the corpus luteum. What we have heard is only information which suggests that in the presence of corpus luteum-insufficiency reproductive function is not completely normal. If, however, one defines the 'mixed bag' on the basis of a progesterone and non-progesterone defect, it is not unusual to use simply progesterone supplementation and have normal implantation and a continuation of pregnancy, if the corpus luteum itself is unessential.

Prof. Rothchild has referred to some controversial baboon work in which the corpus luteum was removed on ideal day 28 of the cycle, and two of four baboons continued on, to deliver little baboons. We agreed that in the human this type of information is not available, yet I have not heard that the corpus luteum is essential for the continuation of early pregnancy. We know that progesterone supplementation after that time is essential. So again, I would think if we are trying to benefit the patients, the direct route of treatment is to the target organ. If we can find the reason that the target organ is inappropriately responding, the mode of treatment should be selected accordingly, but progesterone supplementation should be used as a first attempt before one goes on to a great deal of manipulation of endogenous hormone values using a number of poorly chosen therapies.

Throughout the years it has been shown that if progesterone supplementation for luteal phase insufficiency was begun after the missed menses or, stated differently, when implantation has begun, it does not result in an improvement in pregnancy outcome. The progesterone supplementation must be initiated as early as physiologically possible during the luteal phase. This suggests that the implantation site is what is most important, and everything depends on it having a good start. I have been interested to see that some of us are beginning to agree on the endometrium's importance, but no-one has yet come to a conclusion about how to diagnose what is wrong with that silly corpus luteum, and what to do about it.

189

Insler We really should differentiate between corpus luteum insufficiency as an insufficiency of an organ located in the ovary, and an inappropriate reaction of the endometrium, because otherwise we will be confused.

To call a corpus luteum insufficiency some entity which we diagnose on the basis of an endometrial biopsy only would be terribly wrong. There are reports on endometria with a progesterone receptor deficiency. In such a case the corpus luteum may be perfectly normal. So I think we should distinguish in our discussion two separate entities: a genuine insufficiency of the corpus luteum which should be documented by an inadequate secretion of estrogen and progesterone, and the histological appearance of the endometrium. The latter may or may not be a reflection of the abnormal steroid hormone secretion pattern.

Wentz This is why I was very careful to make the title of my presentation 'luteal phase insufficiency'. I was initially asked to talk about progesterone supplementation of the inadequate corpus luteum, but changed the title. I think we probably do have two entities, but the common denominator is at the level of the endometrium.

Schneider Prof. Rothchild mentioned earlier that a factor which brings about an interaction between the blastocyst and the endometrium could be responsible for the fact that the corpus luteum of pregnancy produces at a very early stage more progesterone than the corpus luteum of non-fertile cycles. I remember that the progesterone production rate rose significantly within 24 hours after ovulation.

Rothchild What you are speaking of is the early pregnancy factor which is measured by some peculiar immunological response. It is, however, not responsible for the change in progesterone secretion which is associated with the interaction of the blastocyst and the endometrium. When I compared the situation in the human, other primates and other mammals, I was impressed by the fact that in almost any instance, except in marsupials, where the pregnancy really does not depend on the corpus luteum except in the very earliest stages, the primary effect of the blastocyst on the corpus luteum is to bring about an abortion of the regression phase in the life-span of the corpus luteum. Superimposed on this may be other patterns of progesterone secretion, but unless that interaction takes place, pregnancy cannot be established.

Insler This factor has to come from the blastocyst rather than the endometrium, otherwise there would have to be a prolonged corpus luteum insufficiency in every case of ectopic pregnancy.

Rothchild The uterus is a very peculiar organ. Even though it is not the only organ in which pregnancy can take place, it is the only one which requires progesterone for that purpose. Very beautiful experiments have been done a long time ago showing that the blastocyst will implant even in a male rat which does not have progesterone or a uterus. When a pregnancy occurs at an ectopic site, it does not need progesterone. The endometrium requires progesterone in a very interesting way, in that it prepares the endometrium for implantation but inhibits the latter. It is only when this inhibition is temporarily blocked by some factor coming from the blastocyst, in some animals it is estrogen, in others it is prostaglandin – the common denominator probably being the prostaglandin effect – that the blastocyst can attach. Consequently, progesterone is important for pregnancy because it occurs in the uterus.

Schneider The question is whether this factor is produced by the blastocyst or not, and if it affects the production rate of progesterone by the corpus luteum?

Wentz An increase in progesterone output has been demonstrated to occur 72 hours after transfer of a cleaved embryo. It is difficult to determine accurately when implantation begins after IVF and embryo transfer, but if we assume that it begins 72 hours later what I am going to say is at least reasonable. I wonder if the progesterone output which occurs from the

190

corpus luteum before this accentuation is essential for the beginning of implantation. Once implantation is proceeding in a relatively normal manner, this cross-talk is established. But I wonder if there ought not to be something in the endometrium too, which is essential for this to occur? This would explain what we all know may happen, the rescue of an inadequate corpus luteum by an early pregnancy. We have all diagnosed corpus luteum inadequacy in patients who treated themselves by becoming pregnant, and lived happily ever after.

One could explain such a rescue situation if the endometrium were capable of taking up the blastocyst, thus allowing the first stages of implantation to occur.

Schneider   As time is running short we should attempt to come to a conclusion on the subject of pathogenesis.

Braendle   I found it very interesting that Prof. Insler succeeded in inducing pregnancies by treatment with LH-RH since we failed at that. One important aspect seems to be that we could not overcome the endogenous rhythm of LH-RH. We have measured the spontaneous fluctuation of FSH and LH during the early follicular phase of normal cycles, anovulatory cycles, and cycles with luteal phase defect, respectively. A lower FSH/LH ratio was found in anovulatory cycles, and those with luteal phase defect when compared to normal cycles. In normal cycles the LH pulsatile pattern showed a typical shift from pulses with low frequency to high frequency during the follicular phase. This shift was lacking in pathological cycles in that a high-frequency pattern of LH fluctuation was already demonstrable during the first days of the follicular phase. Irregularities were noted to occur, too. These alterations were believed to be the result of the missing progesterone effect, as the supplementation with progestins brought about a diminution in the frequency of the LH pulses and a decrease in the mean LH levels.

There are other factors which could be shown to influence the LH fluctuation pattern. In a patient with adrenogenital syndrome the FSH/LH ratio was significantly lower (1/6) and pulsatile pattern irregular with low amplitudes ($\Delta 5$) when the supplementation with cortisol was inadequate, as compared to a phase with adequate supplementation when the FSH/LH ratio rose to 4.5/8, and regular pulses with an amplitude of $\Delta 10$ were demonstrable.

In order to determine if a deficiency of FSH during the early follicular phase may be responsible for the development of a corpus luteum defect, a supplementation with FSH was carried out during the first days of the cycle (150–300 I.U. FSH/day i.m.). As the study is still in progress it would be premature to come to any conclusions, but as yet restoration of normal follicular development and a sufficient luteal phase has not been achieved.

Taubert   In order to reach some sort of consensus on the problem of diagnosis, I would like to propose that we speak of *endometrial inadequacy* if we base the diagnosis on the evaluation of an endometrial biopsy. This may or may not be caused by *luteal inadequacy*, and this should be demonstrated by the measurement of progesterone in an appropriate manner.

Schneider   Do you agree with such a definition?

Bettendorf   I think we could come to an agreement, but what do we imply with the term 'insufficiency'? We are speaking about two organs, the ovary and the endometrium. Ovarian insufficiency can be of follicular or luteal origin, and we have ways to determine this by measuring what makes the follicle or the corpus luteum insufficient with respect to the endometrium. Contrary to that we cannot delineate the function of the endometrium even though the histologists can demonstrate structural changes. I would therefore like to reiterate that luteal phase insufficiency is not a pathognomonic entity but one of many types of ovarian insufficiency. Consequently, we should characterize it like other variants of disturbed ovarian function by considering all diagnostic parameters which could play a role such as LH, FSH, the pulsatile pattern of their release, androgens, prolactin, and finally thyroid values. The endometrial factors have to be evaluated in a different manner. As we did not hear anything new about the existence of a primary endometrial defect, e.g. an endometrium not responding to stimulation by a normally functioning corpus luteum, it will be the task of the histologists to investigate whether or not such an entity plays a significant role.

Schneider What term would you propose we use?

Bettendorf I would prefer to speak about *ovarian insufficiency*.

Breckwoldt May I suggest the term 'insufficient cycle', incompatible with normal pregnancy.

Taubert Those of us working in Germany would have to translate that into German. This would be very difficult with the term suggested by Dr Breckwoldt.

Insler I can hardly agree with Dr Bettendorf, as ovarian insufficiency might also be used to label a case of Turner's syndrome, or some other type of amenorrhoea.

Bettendorf I thought this would have been clear from the beginning, but let me start over again. A patient with disturbed ovarian function will be amenorrhoeic when the estrogens are low, while others bleed spontaneously but do not become pregnant. In the latter group we have to differentiate between patients who have anovulatory cycles, and those in whom we find a progesterone effect in the second part of the cycle. In this group you will find what Dr Breckwoldt and we prefer to call insufficient cycle.

Insler I think what Dr Bettendorf proposes is actually an extension of the WHO-Classification. There is, however, a problem in that the WHO-Classification is therapy-oriented, and is therefore only good for choosing therapy. This is clearly not the case here. I am not a revolutionary; therefore I would rather adhere to the term of *corpus luteum insufficiency* until we have something better.

Schneider Dr Koninckx suggested in his presentation that we speak of the syndrome of corpus luteum insufficiency rather than corpus luteum insufficiency as such.

Koninckx We should not forget that the corpus luteum is secreting a lot more hormones than just progesterone, and their role has not yet been elucidated. Similarly, we know very little about the function of steroid receptors other than progesterone and estrogens in the genesis of the endometrial defect. That is the reason why I would prefer to retain the label of a syndrome of luteal phase defect which encompasses many facets but permits us to define specific causes. I would also like to comment shortly on the problem of anovulatory conditions. Prof. Robertson of London, who is at this moment about 65 years of age, has stated that he never saw in his whole life an oocyte in curettings of the endometrium. He implied, out of this observation, that anovulation may be more prevalent than commonly believed.

Schweppe We are dealing with a group of patients who by definition have a progesterone deficit in the luteal phase. If we subtract cases of endometrial insufficiency, ovulatory disturbances, follicular phase disturbances, and disturbed hypothalamo-pituitary function, we are left with the patient having a defective corpus luteum. But what characterizes such a case?

Schneider This leads back to my previous question whether the release of an ovum is compatible with corpus luteum insufficiency.

Rothchild I think that this is so, even though it is hard to prove. I pointed out before that the whole complex is not peculiar to humans but occurs in other animals, and in those it has been shown that a corpus luteum which secretes less than normal amounts of progesterone can be associated with ovulation as demonstrated by a stigma, and the extrusion of an oocyte from the follicle.

Schneider	Which possibilities do we have to mimic corpus luteum insufficiency other than the use of clomiphene and indomethacin.
Rothchild	Another approach would be the treatment of female monkeys with female inhibin. The point which comes out of this is that there are probably a great many causes. One should state, just because Hodgen induced the formation of an inadequate corpus luteum with female inhibin, that female inhibin or a low FSH level are the only causes. We should not try to be too specific at this point.
Schneider	I would like to summarize what has so far been suggested for naming this entity: ovarian insufficiency, insufficient cycle, corpus luteum insufficiency, syndrome of luteal phase defect, and luteal phase defect.
Rothchild	Luteal phase defect, 'LPD', is a very convenient abbreviation which we have been using all along.
Runnebaum	This term definitely needs some interpretation. Do we really have criteria for the assumption that there is a defect in the corpus luteum?
Rothchild	There is not only early follicular phase-related LPD, but there is also luteal phase-related LPD, and mid-cycle-related LPD. LPD includes all this, and is therefore a very convenient term in that it does not specify the cause.
Schneider	It seems that LPD is the term of choice.
Wentz	The question was asked whether there is any morphological determinant at the ovarian level which can be correlated with other definitions of luteal phase defect. In 1970 Georgeanna Seegar Jones published a study (*Am. J. Obstet. Gynecol.* **108**: 847) in which gonadotropins, urinary pregnanediol, and estrogens were correlated with ovarian morphology in volunteers who agreed to undergo ovarian biopsy of the corpus luteum following clomiphene therapy. What Dr Jones demonstrated, in brief, was as follows: when the stimulation by FSH was inadequate, the corpus luteum at biopsy showed an insufficient granulosa cell layer. In a cycle characterized by a very low LH surge there was no stigma formation, and the ovum remained entrapped within the corpus luteum. Finally, poor stimulation by LH, both during the pre-ovulatory and luteal phase, was shown to result in equally poor theca luteinization. Therefore, one does have some morphological correlates with hormonal data. Unfortunately, at least in the United States, the study can never be repeated, and so I think we have to fall back on what we can learn from old information.
Schneider	As we really should try to cover at least some of the diagnostic and therapeutic aspects in the remaining time, I would like to ask what you consider as the basic requirements for adequate diagnosis in clinical practice?
Insler	If you are talking about establishing the diagnosis in a large number of patients, I think the BBT, progesterone, and the endometrial biopsy would be sufficient. In a clinical research project, however, daily measurements of steroid hormones would be essential, eventually complemented by an endometrial biopsy.
Schneider	You failed to mention ultrasound!
Insler	I did not, as our group is not yet in a position to recognize with certainty a corpus luteum.
Schneider	I would like to summarize that everybody seems to be in agreement that the diagnosis should be based on the BBT, progesterone measurements, and the endometrial biopsy.
Taubert	I wondered why more has not been said about monitoring luteal function by the measurement of progesterone and estradiol. The question remains to be answered as to when, and how many times, progesterone should be determined to evaluate corpus luteum function.
Insler	I think that at least two samples should be obtained 2–3 days apart, and between the 5th and 10th day of the hyperthermic phase of the BBT. This is quite simple to do. I would like to add that in those cycles in which we also determined estradiol, we could not find any special change in the estradiol/progesterone ratio.

Lehmann I think that we should include more criteria in the basic diagnostic work-up than just the BBT, two or three progesterone samples and, maybe, the endometrial biopsy. One should also follow the development of the follicle, its increase in diameter from day to day, particularly during that period in which the largest diameter will be reached. If you find a patient to have a follicle of 12 mm diameter, it suffices to see her again after 4 days, when the crucial stage is reached. Beginning at this stage, estradiol should also be determined daily.

Wentz We have maintained over the years an evaluation that has looked at: (1) the male factor by seminalysis, (2) the mucus factor by starting with the postcoital test, (3) the tubal factor with the hysterosalpingogram, and (4) by doing an endometrial biopsy all in the first cycle of evaluation. This gives us information on five of the six basic infertility factors: ovulatory, male, mucus, endometrial, and tubal. After a wait of 3 months a diagnostic laparoscopy is done. The importance of the endometrial biopsy is that it is relatively inexpensive as compared to multiple hormone determinations; it does not fail to detect entities which will be missed by single, double, or triple hormone measurements; and it is something which will at least provide something approaching a bioassay of corpus luteum function.

Rothchild I do not expect that two or even three progesterone levels are going to be an answer because of the pattern which we saw. The reliability of the AUC depends very much on the overall pattern, and that makes its clinical application almost impossible. If the endometrial biopsy yields information which says there is nothing wrong with the endometrium, there is really no point in following up with progesterone determinations. What is important is if the endometrium is out-of-phase or defective in some other way. Then one is obligated to demonstrate whether this is associated with normal or abnormal progesterone levels. If the progesterone levels are normal, it is obvious that progesterone administration is not the treatment of choice. When the endometrium in the presence of normal progesterone levels is defective, there is something wrong with the endometrial response, and this is what has to be looked for. But if the progesterone level is abnormal, one can logically treat with progesterone. At this point one can decide how many times, and at what time of the cycle, one can get the most reliable information about progesterone. I would like to point out that there are RIAs for progesterone some of which are not as specific as the kind we would use at a research laboratory. They are, however, adequate for the clinical situation, and are easy to use.

Breckwoldt The observation of the cervical mucus is also of value for the timing of ultrasound examinations. When we see that there is an increase of secretion we subject the patient to sonography in order to determine the diameter of the leading follicle. Whenever there is a leading follicle of more than 12 mm in diameter we can calculate the further development by the growth velocity, which is about 2.5 mm per day.

Daume I fully concur with Dr Breckwoldt in that it is possible in most of these cases to demonstrate the collapse of the follicle.

Lehmann It has to be emphasized that it is mandatory to have such equipment available if an Infertility Centre is to treat patients in this category. This statement should, however, not be misunderstood. I did not advocate this type of intensive follow-up as a matter of routine, but it should be used for the benefit of those patients who show signs of this syndrome.

Schneider Did you mean to say that the use of ultrasound is obligatory in the diagnosis of luteal phase inadequacy?

Lehmann Yes, I did.

Bettendorf I would like to bring two very simple diagnostic tools to your attention: the cervical mucus and the basal body temperature, the use of which should not be abandoned altogether in favour of more sophisticated methods. Whenever the cervical mucus fails to undergo the typical changes within

	2 days after ovulation, it is very likely that there is something wrong with the corpus luteum. The same applies to the increase of the BBT following ovulation.
Köhler	I would like to comment on the statement of Prof. Rothchild that an endometrial defect must be present if progesterone levels are normal, and the endometrium is out-of-phase. The histological appearance of the endometrium may in fact be due to a hormonal aberration which occurred in a previous cycle, and endometrial rests which have not properly been shed may actually interfere with implantation.
Schneider	That leads one to the question as to how long you ought to administer therapy to rid the endometrium of such incompletely shed remnants carried over from an insufficient cycle?
Wentz	That could only be asserted if you perform a biopsy on day 5 of cycle. Having read every biopsy for the past 15 years, I have not seen that, however.
Schweppe	I agree with you that you would have to do a biopsy in the early follicular phase of the following cycle. Our argument was, however, based on ultrastructural findings. The high number of electro-light cells showing various degrees of disorganization and differentiation could be explained by such a mechanism.
Dallenbach-Hellweg	There is histological evidence that the endometrium is not shed completely in certain pathological conditions. Even in normal cycles it sometimes fails to do that, the extreme being what we call silent menstruation. In cases of irregular shedding we find star-shaped glands and large areas of regenerating endometrial glands on day 10 of the cycle, which are ultimately incorporated into the endometrium of the new cycle. There is indeed reason to rid the endometrium of such remnants.
Wentz	The point was made that you cannot recognize that when you do a biopsy late in the luteal phase. In order to do that by means of light-microscopy you would have to perform the biopsy in the proliferative phase!
Dallenbach-Hellweg	I agree with that.
Rothchild	I have the impression that we are confounding two things. Most of the people present here are engaged in research, and we have to distinguish between research purposes and clinical interests. If we are dealing with a routine clinical situation, we should follow the suggestions made by Dr Wentz. I do not think, however, that there is a place for the measurement of progesterone unless you want to establish a real curve. The same applies to the use of ultrasound, which in the near future will probably be proven to be a powerful diagnostic tool.
Schneider	My personal impression is that at the moment the specialists in the audience prefer to employ whatever diagnostic tool they command. It will, therefore, be very difficult to arrive at some consensus on how to economize. Everybody will have to decide that for himself. Moreover, we have to move on to the discussion of therapeutic aspects.
Koninckx	First, I would like to support the plea made for progesterone supplementation as a first approach to therapy. Thereafter, I want to add two points on the use of clomiphene. We have re-viewed the cases of 200 patients who received clomiphene therapy for the past 10 years. Two factors evolved, the observation of which appears to be essential for the success of this type of therapy. In the first treatment cycle there were about 5% pregnancies. In the second cycle of treatment another 15% of patients conceived, and this difference was significant. After the second treatment cycle there was one cycle without therapy, and in this cycle 12% of the patients became pregnant. This leads to the conclusion that clomiphene is not only effective in the cycle of administration, but that this effect carries over into the subsequent cycle. This beneficial effect could possibly be explained by the observations made by Dr Schweppe and his co-workers on retained endometrial remnants.

195

Schneider If you consider clomiphene treatment as a second approach to therapy, for what period of time should it be used, would you eventually increase the dose, and would you recommend treatment-free intervals? Finally, what would you do if this fails, too?

Koninckx It is difficult to answer these questions on the basis of statistics. If you are dealing with a situation in which you can expect a pregnancy rate of 5–10% per cycle, and you want to achieve a pregnancy rate of approximately 90%, you have to administer treatment for 2 years, and I think nobody is willing to do that.

Insler We should also take into consideration the fact that the majority of clomiphene-induced pregnancies occurs within the first six treatment cycles. To continue treatment beyond that period of time requires at least a re-evaluation and a restatement of the unchanged necessity for this treatment. Incidentally, we administer clomiphene in alternating cycles only, and there are almost as many pregnancies in the treatment-free cycles as in treatment cycles. This supports the notion on the incorporation of endometrium from a previous cycle into that of the following one.

Schneider This is an observation which I can fully confirm. Moreover, the therapeutic effect of clomiphene may also be carried over into the next one by promoting follicular maturation and the recruitment of the future dominant follicle in the regression phase of the treatment cycle.

Rothchild It has been shown a long time ago, and it has been confirmed by the work of Hodgen and co-workers in the monkey, that it takes about 2 weeks for a small antral follicle to reach the size of pre-ovulation.

Schneider This is also the time of the cycle in which the LH-pulse rate increases stepwise from approximately one pulse in every 6 hours to about four pulses. There is only a very discrete rise in serum FSH following this variation in frequency of pulsatility, and it has been argued that it is very often not possible to confirm by statistics whether the rising FSH level is responsible for the recruitment of the leading follicle. The question is really if we should not consider starting treatment already in the late luteal phase of the preceding cycle in order to promote folliculogenesis for the succeeding cycle, rather than having patients take an ovulation-inducing agent beginning on day 5 of the cycle, as the selection of the dominant follicle occurs already on day 6 or 7.

Rothchild I do not know whether clomiphene treatment works in other ways, too, because we are so used to doing it this way. The reason for this goes back to the early days of clomiphene therapy when one wanted to make sure that the patient had menstruated before beginning treatment. Since menstruation usually lasts for 5 days, and the first day of menstruation is considered as the first day of the cycle, it has become a practice to start clomiphene treatment on day 5. When the patient is not menstruating, or when we are trying to change the pattern of follicular growth, it probably would be physiologically better to start on day 1.

Schneider As it has been pointed out by Dr Yen that the negative feedback effect is best expressed on day 5 of the cycle, the anti-estrogen effect should be most effective at this time.

Rothchild That is not the only point. The effectiveness of clomiphene comes from its ability to inhibit the inhibiting activity of estrogens on gonadotropin secretion. During the time clomiphene is given the gonadotropins are rising, but its effectiveness does not manifest itself during the time of treatment but in the period following treatment.

Schneider How about starting treatment late in the luteal phase?

Rothchild I do not know but it would be worth a try.

Lehmann It has been shown in IVF programmes that the number of degenerated oocytes increases with the number of cycles clomiphene is given. After three or four continuous cycles of treatment, the percentage of degenerated oocytes approaches 40–50%. This is a fact we were not aware of before the advent of IVF. We should take these data into consideration and apply clomiphene no longer in an uninterrupted manner.

Bettendorf
We made a similar observation in spontaneously bleeding patients treated with hMG, that the pregnancy rate was greater when treatment was administered in an intermittent rather than a continuous fashion. When clomiphene became available we used to start treatment on day 7 of the cycle but noticed that ovulation occurred often rather late. As a consequence, we went back to day 5, and finally to day 3 which appears to mimic the normal ovarian cycle much better.

Wentz
A comment concerning biopsies. We have found that a second biopsy is essential to make the diagnosis of luteal phase insufficiency, and I would reiterate that. Without a second biopsy there will be a tendency to overdiagnose a very rare condition. I would disagree that this biopsy can be taken after menstruation has begun, for two reasons. An intact capsule is, in our hands, essential for the diagnosis and evaluation of the decidual reaction. A disruption of the capsule prevents one from determining this effect. We have also not found any increase in miscarriage rate or any other untoward effect upon pregnancy by biopsies taken in the cycle of conception. And I would of course agree with you that a biopsy should be taken in the cycle of therapy to see if something is being done. Coming back to your comment concerning clomiphene: when clomiphene is begun on day 3 one finds that actually fewer follicles are being recruited and fewer oocytes are obtained. If one begins clomiphene on day 5 or 6 of the cycle, one obtains more developed follicles and more oocytes, which is really not in contrast to what has been said. What you see is actually the initiation of the LH surge about 11–12 days after the onset of clomiphene administration, no matter when it is given, day 2, 3, or 6. So it seems to be the day of clomiphene administration which starts the ball rolling. We achieved a better pregnancy rate when we started on day 5; the reason being that we see less of an anti-estrogenic effect.

Insler
There must be a difference between spontaneous and stimulated cycles because Hodgen showed in the monkey that you can obtain a new crop of follicles by continuous stimulation. The follicles eventually undergo atresia, but if you continue with hMG, you will have a new crop.

Rothchild
There is some interesting information on that. In the rat, for example, there are two waves of FSH: one just at the time of the LH surge, and another very short one, about a day later. The second one is important for recruiting the follicles that will result in ovulation in the following cycle. The information which we obtain from clomiphene treatment of people, and the kind of information which Hodgen obtained by removing the dominant follicle, all that adds up to a picture of a certain time requirement for a follicle to develop from the early antral stage to ovulation. If that answer is correct, under conditions in which the secretion of gonadotropins has been changed by the effects of clomiphene, for example, this process can be shortened considerably. The 17-day interval which you mentioned is very consistent, but yet the effect of clomiphene indicates that this process can be shortened down to almost less than a week, because you have to consider the time from the last administration of clomiphene to the time of the LH surge. In anovulatory patients this tends to be about a week and a half. In the patient who is ovulating regularly, when you start treatment on day 5 there will be an ovulation still at the expected time. The time for follicular development is obviously shortened.

Insler
Just consider the Group Ia amenorrhoea patients treated with hMG; it does not take 17 days until ovulation occurs, and you start with an quiescent ovary. This proves that there is a difference between treatment cycles and spontaneous cycles.

Schneider
Time is running short! Even though treatment with hMG and clomiphene has been thoroughly covered, bromocriptine and LH-RH have not yet been mentioned.

Insler I do not think that LH-RH is a good choice of treatment for spontaneously menstruating women, as these patients with luteal phase inadequacy are. We tried it for the purpose of proving that induction of ovulation may correct the luteal defect, but there was no advantage over clomiphene.

Schneider It has been proposed to render a patient amenorrhoeic and to start a new cycle thereafter.

Bettendorf We tried this once; i.e. to block ovulation in one cycle and to stimulate it in the following, but it did not seem to improve matters much.

L'Hermite I would like to comment on your proposition to block ovulation and administer gonadotropins. There has been a report from the group of Coutts, which looked quite interesting. They desensitized the hypo-thalamo-pituitary–ovarian axis with the aid of a potent LH-RH analogue, and then, after about 15 days, while maintaining this treatment, stimulated the ovaries with gonadotropins. As far as can be judged from the first report, in cases of unexplained infertility and luteal defect they seem to have obtained quite a nice pregnancy rate.

Rothchild Do I have the last word? I think the last word should be said with something that was said a long time ago by Axel Westmann of Sweden. In an examination of all the possible causes of infertility and associated dis-orders, he made the very important point that regardless of any form of treatment, or even with no treatment at all, about 30–35% of the patients get better by themselves. We do not always remember this, but any method of treatment has to be measured against the possibility that the spon-taneous rate is somewhat in the neighborhood of 1 out of every 3 patients.

Schneider This was a very appropriate statement for concluding this session, and with that I would like to turn over the chair to our scientific secretary.

Taubert The battle is over, the heroes are tired, but the issues remain, even though some of them may appear less clouded than before, when we set out to unravel the mysteries of the inadequate luteal phase. The concentration on such a narrow issue proved to have been the right move, as far as can be judged from the lively discussion. I would like to thank all of you for making this workshop possible, especially the speakers for the preparation of their manuscripts, and the chairpersons for guiding the discussion along the right channels. Finally, I am sure I express your sentiments when I ask Mr Felbier and Dr Musil to accept our sincere thanks to Serono of Germany for sponsoring this workshop as the VIIth Freiburg Colloquium.

Editors' Comment

H.-D. TAUBERT AND H. KUHL

The common denominator of this workshop was a growing perception that the pathogenesis of luteal phase inadequacy is even more complex than it could reasonably be expected. Even though there was unequivocal agreement among the members of this panel that the causes of luteal phase inadequacy are manifold, no consensus could be reached on the question of which hormonal, metabolic, or morphological criteria, apart from the measurement of progesterone and the endometrial biopsy, seem to be of particular clinical value. The lack of agreement over the meaning of diagnostic features was reflected by the inconclusive end to the deliberations on how to name this elusive cause of infertility in lieu of a term which would clearly designate its cause.

The functional capacity of the corpus luteum is without doubt determined by the maturation of follicles well in advance of ovulation, and possibly by a number of periovulatory events. The intricate synergisms of FSH and LH in the regulation of steroid synthesis by the theca and granulosa means that subtle deviations from the normal pattern of gonadotropin release may disturb follicular maturation. It is, therefore, conceivable that the close interrelationship between the feedback mechanisms within the hypothalamo-pituitary-ovarian axis could possibly contribute to an intensification of actually minor disturbances. An FSH deficiency during the early follicular phase, for example, may result in a reduction of aromatase activity, and thus impair estrogen production. Similarly, an LH deficiency may affect follicular development adversely in that inadequate amounts of androgens are provided as precursors of estrogen synthesis. Conversely, follicular development can be retarded in the presence of excessive amounts of LH, and this may result in atresia. When the disorder is characterized by elevated testosterone levels, there is a direct relationship between this and the length of the luteal phase (Smith *et al., Fertil. Steril.*, **32** (1979), 403). This leads to the conclusion that the maintenance of a normal ratio between FSH and LH throughout the phase of follicular development is an essential prerequisite for the formation of a normal corpus luteum.

The association between hyperprolactinaemia and defective follicular development and formation of an inadequate corpus luteum remains to be a subject of some controversy – at least with respect to eventual therapeutic consequences. Luteal phase inadequacy does not seem to be caused in such cases by a direct effect of excessive amounts of prolactin upon the ovary, but rather by a disturbance at the level of the hypothalamus and the pituitary.

Ovulation and transformation of the collapsed follicle into a sufficiently functioning corpus luteum depend also on an appropriate LH surge, and the latter is at least partly governed by the rising levels of estradiol reflecting follicular maturation. There is growing evidence that the ovulatory process is not an 'all-or-nothing-phenomenon', in that disturbances of various degrees of severity may either cause anovulation without signs of luteinization, retention of the oocyte within a luteinized, unruptured follicle which may hormonally mimick a normal corpus luteum, or inadequate luteal function subsequent to the release of the oocyte.

Luteal phase inadequacy may also manifest itself at the target organ of progesterone, the endometrium. Adequate secretory transformation of a sufficiently proliferated endometrium depends on a balanced and well-timed interaction of estradiol and progesterone which is mediated by the respective receptors. Both the estradiol and progesterone receptor reach the highest concentration shortly before ovulation, and this is followed by a decrease to a nadir on day 22 of the cycle. It is noteworthy that there is no correlation between the serum levels of estradiol and progesterone, and the concentration of the receptors in the endometrium during the secretory phase of a normal cycle. This discrepancy is probably brought about by intrinsic endometrial factors such as a progesterone-stimulated increase in endometrial 17β-hydroxy-steroid dehydrogenase activity, resulting in a rapid metabolization of estradiol.

The inadequate and normal secretory endometrium do not differ much with respect to the concentration of both the nuclear and cytoplasmic progesterone receptor. In contrast to this, the endometrium of luteal phase inadequacy has been shown to contain less estradiol receptor as a normal secretory endometrium, possibly due to an impairment of estradiol secretion during the pre-ovulatory period (Levy et al., Am. J. Obstet. Gynecol., **136**, (1980), 646). A certain level of estradiol appears to be an essential factor for normophasic endometrial maturation, but excessive amounts of estradiol can interfere with the action of progesterone.

The present state of knowledge concerning the pathogenesis of luteal phase inadequacy can be summarized by stating that the cause or causes of this entity remain uncertain, as it is very likely that some, as yet unknown, factors are involved. Therefore, it did not come as a surprise that all attempts to diagnose this entity by a more specific test than the endometrial biopsy or by steroid measurements in serum have failed so far, and the endeavour to develop such tests seems to have reached a certain impass.

It would appear to be practical to distinguish between *luteal inadequacy* and *endometrial inadequacy* in clinical practice. The former can as yet only be demonstrated by the measurement of progesterone and possibly estradiol in blood, but no real agreement could be reached on the question as to how to proceed in clinical practice, although the potential usefulness of ultrasound for identifying an abnormal corpus luteum was generally accepted.

Endometrial inadequacy can only be proven by a well-timed biopsy. It should, however, be kept in mind that neither progesterone measurements nor the endometrial biopsy can be used to predict each other (Shangold *et al., Fertil. Steril.*, **40**, (627), 1983), as an endometrial defect can exist in the presence of a normally functioning corpus luteum. The examination of endometrial specimens by means of electron microscopy or histochemistry, assay of endometrial prolactin production, or the measurement of the steroid receptor content in the endometrium has not yet reached a stage of development which would justify the introduction of one or the other of these methods into the clinical routine.

When the diagnosis of luteal or endometrial inadequacy or of both has been established beyond doubt, a search for the underlying cause or causes such as alterations in the secretory pattern of gonadotropins, prolactin, androgens, and the thyroid hormones should be considered on an individual basis, even though the discussion at this workshop clearly showed that it is not yet possible to supply universally applicable guide-lines for doing this.

The clinician trying to diagnose and treat luteal phase inadequacy has to be cognisant of the fact that luteal phase inadequacy

- does not have to be a constant phenomenon,
- may undergo spontaneous remission,
- does not have to be incompatible with pregnancy, as a process of self-healing may be initiated after conception,
- may only be one facet out of a wide spectrum of ovarian dysfunction which also includes anovulation, the LUF-syndrome, and occasionally normal cycles.

As the presently available diagnostic tools can entail considerable expense to the patient in most countries, a calculation of the cost-to-benefit ratio comparing a simplistic approach, limited, for example, to the use of the basal body temperature record and the endometrial biopsy, to a highly sophisticated one should not be considered as pure heresy.

The ambivalence with respect to diagnostics found a counterpart in the discussion of therapeutic aspects in that there is obviously no really good indicator which one could depend on in order to choose between substitution with progesterone during the luteal phase or stimulation with hMG or clomiphene during the follicular phase. The substitution with progesterone may improve the endocrine milieu in the endometrium and thus promote implantation. In addition, the beneficial effect of progesterone may be extended into the following cycle by promoting complete shedding of the endometrium which will result in better conditions for implantation. It has, however, also been demonstrated that a pregnancy can develop in an out-of-phase endometrium. This observation raises some doubts on the efficacy of hormonal treatment of luteal phase inadequacy.

There was general consent that the pregnancy rate in patients with luteal phase inadequacy is lower than in patients with anovulation, and that the results do not differ much with respect to modes of treatment or even the absence of treatment. When ovulation has been demonstrated beyond doubt, e.g. by laparoscopy and a high progesterone gradient between the peritoneal fluid and serum, or is at least very likely, treatment with progesterone appears to be justified. Emphasis was placed on the use of progesterone by the vaginal route, as not all synthetic progestogens seem to be capable of duplicating the biological effects of the natural compound, and there remains some concern as to possible teratogenic effects.

As the functional development of the ovum predetermines the ultimate success of fertilization and implantation to a large degree, the therapeutic efforts should be focussed in the remaining patients on promoting follicular development. Although hMG, clomiphene, and, to a lesser degree, LH-RH, have been shown to be effective in the treatment of luteal phase inadequacy, the preference for one or other of these agents should at the present time be guided by the personal experience of the physician, as it became apparent from the discussion that there are as yet no large-scale prospective studies demonstrating one of these therapeutic agents to be superior to any other.

The observation that pregnancies occur in cycles of biopsy showing endometrial inadequacy could certainly lead into therapeutic nihilism. When contemplating the possible causes of luteal phase inadequacy, however, in a more positive way, it must be concluded that even though this workshop did not provide ready-made solutions as to how to diagnose and treat luteal phase inadequacy better than before, it succeeded in making us aware that the investigation of luteal phase inadequacy offers a unique access to a better understanding of the immensely complex interactions within the reproductive system and its disturbances.

Index

203